To AUDREY
with love
John.
1998 - 10 - 5

CANADIAN MEDICAL LIVES

LEONARD ALBERT MILLER

Public Servant

John R. Martin

Series Editor: T.P. Morley, M.D.

Associated Medical Services, Incorporated
and
Fitzhenry & Whiteside

Fitzhenry & Whiteside
195 Allstate Parkway
Markham, Ontario L3R 4T8

Book Design: Darrell McCalla

Printing and Binding: University of Toronto Press Inc.

Fitzhenry & Whiteside wishes to acknowledge the generous assistance and ongoing support of The Book Publishing Industry Development Programme of Heritage Canada.

Canadian Cataloguing in Publications Data

Martin, John R., 1922-
Leonard Albert Miller, public servant

(Canadian medical lives)
Includes index.

ISBN 1-55041-190-X

1. Miller, Leonard Albert. 2. Medical policy – Newfoundland.
3. Cabinet ministers – Newfoundland – Biography. I. Title.
II. Series.
RA395.C3M375 1998 353.6′2293′09718 C98-930152-4

To Claire

CANADIAN MEDICAL LIVES SERIES

The story of the Hannah Institute for the History of Medicine has been told by John B. Neilson and G.R. Paterson in *Associated Medical Services Incorporated: A History (1987)*. Dr. Donald R. Wilson, then President of AMS, and the Board of directors decided that the Institute should produce this series of biographies as one of its undertakings.

This is the twentieth volume in the series. All these biographies can be obtained through the retail book trade or from Fitzhenry & Whiteside, 195 Allstate Parkway, Markham ON L3R 4T8.

John Martin, a non-governmental medical colleague and long-time friend of Leonard Miller, is well qualified to write the story of Miller (1906-1981) whose career as civil servant in the Newfoundland government probably spanned more continuous years than any senior Canadian public servant. Martin shows how political savvy and trustworthiness in personal relationships together made for his success. Miller was powerful because he was discreet, diplomatic and loyal to his elected superiors, but he did not shrink from giving advice to the most obdurate of politicians when he saw danger ahead.

There is no shortage of meritorious subjects. Willing and capable authors are harder to acquire. AMS is therefore deeply grateful to authors who have committed their time and skill to the series.

T.P. Morley
Series Editor
1998

CANADIAN MEDICAL LIVES SERIES

Duncan Graham by Robert B. Kerr & Douglas Waugh

Bill Mustard by Marilyn Dunlop

Joe Doupe by Terence Moore

Emily Stowe by Mary Beacock Fryer

Clarence Hincks by Charles G. Roland

Francis A.C. Scrimger, V.C., by Suzanne Kingsmill

Earle P. Scarlett by F. W. Musselwhite

R.G. Ferguson by Stuart Houston

Harold Griffith by Richard Bodman & Dierdre Gillies

Maude Abbott by Douglas Waugh

William Boyd by Ian Carr

J.C. Boileau Grant by C. L. N. Robinson

R.M. Bucke by Peter A. Rechnitzer

William Henry Drummond by J.B.Lyons

Alan Brown by A.B. Kingsmill

Harold N. Segall by C.G. Roland

William R. Beaumont by Julian A. Smith

David M. Baltzan by Verne Clemence

Jean I. Gunn by Natalie Riegler

Leonard Albert Miller by John R. Martin

CONTENTS

Acknowledgements

Dr. Nigel Rusted, a contemporary of Miller, provided me with copies of Miller's unpublished memoirs and other writings and was a fund of information on Miller's earlier days. Drs. Ian Rusted and W.D. Parsons, Mrs. Lorraine Balderson, Mrs. Ruby Squires, Mrs. Joan Coates and Mr. Mark Shrimpton kindly put at my disposal letters and other records in their possession. To members of the Miller family, Mrs. Lorraine Balderson, Ms. Yvette Brooks and Mr. Michael Miller, I am indebted for photographs and information on the genealogy of the Miller family.

I am under a deep obligation to the Newfoundland and Labrador Medical Association and especially to the late Mr. Gerald Lynch, the Executive Director, for permission to use the archives of the association and to photostat material at no charge.

The staff of the Provincial Archives of Newfoundland and Labrador and the Centre of Newfoundland Studies have been unfailingly helpful in advice and locating material relevant to Miller's career. Dr. Jean Gray of Dalhousie University kindly provided details on Miller's academic career. Mr. John O'Reilly and other friends have directed my attention to relevant books and records.

I express my thanks to all these people for their assistance and also supplying me with clarification in response to my many inquiries.

Professors John Crellin and Susan McCorquodale reviewed the entire manuscript and Ms. Janet Story, Chapter 19. I am grateful to them for this time-consuming job and their helpful comments. They are of course in no way responsible for the opinions expressed in the book.

Professor Malcolm MacLeod kindly volunteered to compile the index; needless to say I was only too happy to accept his offer, and I am deeply indebted to him for this time-consuming task which he has performed so expertly, with the assistance of Kelly Murrin. Typing the index was handled by Beverly Evans-Hong and Vanessa Rice and I express my thanks to them.

To Mrs. Elizabeth Sheppard, who typed countless revisions of this manuscript, I express my deepest thanks. Finally, my wife Claire, to whom I am dedicating this book, must be thanked for her patience for accepting my obsession with Leonard Miller, proof reading and shrewd comments.

Introduction

"Let every man be swift to hear, slow to speak, slow to wrath" – James 1:19 (AV)

"I have done the state some service" – Othello. Wm. Shakespeare quoted by Dr. G. Story in presenting Dr. Leonard A. Miller for the degree of Doctor of Science (Honoris Causa) 16 October 1971.

These two quotations sum up the character and career of Leonard Albert Miller.

The administrative structures and institutions of the British North American colonies were patterned after those in the UK. Confederation, time and local circumstances have introduced divergences on this side of the Atlantic, but they still bear the imprint of their origins on the civil service.

Miller's formative years were passed under Commission of Government when Newfoundland was governed directly from London. It was then he began his career as a civil servant. It was one of the objects of that government to train a civil service after the model of Whitehall.

What sort of image does a Whitehall civil servant of the 1930s conjure up? He would be patriotic, self-effacing, hardworking, discreet, and incorruptible. But just to have shown these virtues hardly qualifies their possessor to be the subject of a biography. To merit such notice he would have had to be more than a worthy but pedestrian civil servant. He would have had to exhibit unusual traits and to have been outstandingly successful in his field of work.

The aim of this biography is to show that this was true of Miller.

It was as an accomplished and distinguished civil servant that Miller made his mark and for which he is remembered. His career is inextricably linked with the evolution of health services in Newfoundland during the days of Commission of Government (1934-49) and the Smallwood era (1949-1972). In one capacity or another he was involved in the major health care policy decisions of those years and indeed it is the part he played in these events which gives his career significance.

He joined the civil service as a part-time Medical Officer of Health (MHO) in 1933 and then full-time in 1934. In 1944 he was promoted Director of Medical Services, the senior civil servant responsible for the Health Services of the Department of Public Health and Welfare. In 1949, when Newfoundland joined Canada, he became Deputy Minister of Health, a position he held until his retirement in 1971. As Deputy Minister, Miller represented his province on a number of federal/provincial committees and at the meetings of the ministers and deputy ministers of health. Here also, he stood out. So highly was he regarded that on two occasions he was chosen to be one of the Canadian delegates to the World Health Organization.

In some respects Miller lived in fortunate times: he was at the helm of his department during a time of unparalleled prosperity for Newfoundland, the days when governments had money to spend. It was Miller who had to decide which new projects before the government were deserving of financial support. He did not have to face budget cutbacks, downsizing and curtailment of services. It was also before the days of intense media scrutiny. Miller did not have to concern himself about public relations and he was never buttonholed by the press to answer embarrassing questions.

I made the acquaintance of Miller in the early seventies when I was editor of the Newfoundland Medical Association (NMA) Newsletter. I approached him to write an article on the cottage hospitals of Newfoundland. Miller was only too willing to comply. This led to a friendship which lasted to the day he died. Although a newcomer to Newfoundland, I soon sensed that this was a most unusual personage, and like so many others I developed a high regard and affection for him.

A word about the method adopted in writing this biography and the use of terms. The book is the product of archival research and interviews with colleagues and friends who knew or worked with Miller. For statements derived from written records the appropriate references have been supplied. In the case of opinions based on oral testimony, I have adopted the practice frequently of putting these in quotations marks although they may not be exact quotations.

Newfoundland is the legal title for the province of Newfoundland and Labrador and this is the sense in which it is employed in this book. Newfoundland was a self-governing Colony until 1931; then a Dominion; followed by Commission of Government in 1934 and since 1949 a Province of Canada. I use whichever term is appropriate to the period under discussion.

CHAPTER 1

Three Incidents

The Child Welfare Association clinic was bedlam. Distraught mothers were trying to calm screaming babies and infants. Harassed nurses and volunteer workers were at their wits' end. In strode a plump, balding young physician. As if by magic order began to reign. With a soothing word here or a word of warning there to a mother or to a child, calm descended. Soon, in a tranquil atmosphere, he went about his business of examining babies and infants. As one volunteer remembers, "It was like Elvis Presley. He was idolized. He could do anything with mothers or their children. Mothers would ask if he would be coming to the clinic and if the answer was no, they would go away." But children were always his first love. Their needs were always uppermost in his plans and actions. His one and only recorded boast was the spectacular improvement in child health during his days in office.

●

It was an idyllic Newfoundland summer day, one of those days, all too rare, when people long to drop everything and get outdoors to savor every precious minute. Inside, the NMA was holding its annual meeting. This was the final day of the business section. It was now noon. Soon the luncheon would follow at which, as was the custom, the Deputy Minister of Health, Len (as he was known to the doctors) Miller would give his annual state of the union address reviewing the department's accomplishments during the past year and unveiling what it proposed to do in the coming days. At these luncheons he gave the impression that he was passing on confidential information. Nothing of course could have been further from the truth. But the doctors enjoyed the illusion of feeling they had been taken into his confidence. The chairman terminated the morning business and then added that since it was such a beautiful day many members might want to forgo the luncheon and join their spouses on an outing on the river. There were still lots of spaces available on the boats.

Silence. Not a chair scraped the floor. No one got up to escape. The Deputy Minister's famous smile played back and forth on his face. Not a person left the room. Like obedient school children they trooped into a nearby room for lunch and to hear the Deputy Minister of Health. No one would have dared to walk out under his observant eye. Such was the hold he had on the physicians of Newfoundland, an acceptance by the profession that has never been equalled by a Deputy Minister.

●

At a meeting of officials from the federal and provincial departments of health, arguments were heated and as usual were wandering further and further from the point under discussion. The Deputy Minister from Newfoundland had not yet been heard from but now, as was his custom with a little smile, he intervened with a few low-key remarks. "It gave us all a pause and restored perspective," one participant observed. This was Miller's custom. He never spoke early on a point but waited until he thought the psychological moment had come to wrap up the debate. He would then rise to his feet, summarize what had been said, lay out the choices with their pros and cons, indicating which were worth serious attention. Usually his advice was taken, and it was expected that Miller's remarks would be the closing comments in a debate. So high was his reputation among his colleagues across the country that one federal official described him as "the best deputy minister of health in Canada".

CHAPTER 2

The Early Years

When Leonard Albert Miller was born in St. John's on 10 August 1906, Newfoundland was enjoying one of its brief periods of relative prosperity. Sir Robert Bond was the prime minister, one of the few in the colony to leave a reputation of scrupulous honesty. Newfoundland was one of the self-governing colonies of the British Empire, albeit the most sparsely populated and the poorest. The population was only around 220,984 and St. John's, the capital, was a small town of about 29,594*. Miller's formative years and early career were passed in a country that did not become a part of Canada until 1949. It was Newfoundland's unique history that shaped his career.

Newfoundland was discovered by Europeans in the fifteenth century. It was soon realized that its waters were teeming with fish but that the island itself had little to offer for settlement except as a staging post for the offshore fisheries. The European powers vied in exploiting these rich fishing grounds. In 1713 the island was recognized as a British possession by the Treaty of Utrecht. For the next century the history of the island revolved around the fishing merchants of the Dorset coast in England. Each spring they would send out fleets to fish the Newfoundland waters. The catch would be partially salted and dried on land for sale in the Iberian peninsula and Italy. Each autumn the ships would return to England except for

* Census of Newfoundland and Labrador 1901

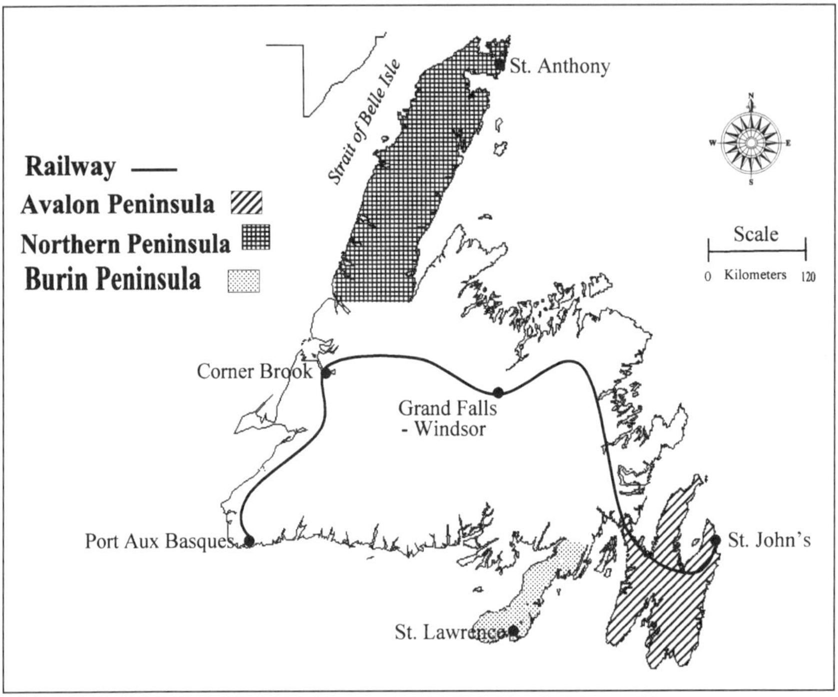

Map of Newfoundland and southern part of Labrador
Courtesy of Mr. D. Gordon, Department of Environment, Government of Newfoundland

those bound for the Mediterranean. The British authorities discouraged permanent settlement but a few small settlements did spring up to take care of gear that had to be left behind and to prepare for the next season's catch. St. John's, as the administrative centre, grew into the largest of the all-year-round establishments.

The exclusive trading era of the coastal merchants of Dorset ended with the French Revolution and the Napoleonic wars which disrupted the itinerant fishing fleets from Europe. For the first time permanent settlements on a modest scale began to spring up. The settlers were transported on boats from the west coast willing to run the risk of capture by French privateers. En route to Newfoundland they would call at Waterford or Wexford in Ireland for provisions and to pick up more settlers. The settlers were made up of those who could walk to Poole in Dorset or Waterford and Wexford. They tended to segregate when they reached Newfoundland, the English settling to the north of St. John's, and the Irish to the south, where to this day they maintain the customs and dialects of their ancestors. The location of their settlements or "outports," as they were called, was dictated by proximity to good fishing grounds and were scattered around coves and on offshore islands. Many were bleak and exposed and in the autumn their inhabitants would migrate to more sheltered locations for the winter months. The settlers continued the pattern of the inshore fisheries, partially salting and drying fish for export to the West Indies and Brazil and, with the conclusion of hostilities in 1815, returning once again to the Mediterranean littoral. The peace also saw the end of immigration on any large scale. A fishing economy then evolved which has been criticized as the bane of Newfoundland. Merchants would supply fishermen with gear and advance supplies and in return fishermen would turn over their catch to the merchants and receive food and other necessities at the merchants' stores. Money rarely changed hands. This method of transacting business, known as "the truck system," dominated the Newfoundland economy until confederation with Canada. Its bad features were the constant indebtedness of the fishermen to the merchants who were able to dictate the value of catches and fix prices at their stores.

In 1855 responsible government was granted. The population was about evenly divided between Protestants and the slightly preponderant Roman Catholics and the economy was almost totally dependent on the fisheries. The government was dominated by the St. John's merchants. The fishermen in the outports, eking out a marginal livelihood, had little interest in who governed them and inevitably power gravitated into the hands of the St. John's merchant oligarchy.

Through its domination of the upper chamber, the crown-appointed legislative council, the merchants controlled the levers of power. Patronage was rampant and distributed on the basis of religious affiliation and party loyalty. Change of government was followed by "spoils to the victor" and the wholesale dismissal of every government employee down to the lowest ranks and their replacement by supporters of the new government. Poverty, with its attendant evils of malnutrition and infectious diseases, was widespread. The St. John's slums were said by one traveller to be the worst she had ever seen. Communications were by boat, and roads were few and in wretched condition. A trans-island railway, linking St. John's with Port-aux -Basques, was completed by 1898 but brought only disappointment and more debts. It did not lead to opening up the interior to development apart from a paper mill at Grand Falls and a mine at Buchans. To this day the interior of the island remains uninhabited. The railway was never solvent and eventually was taken over by the government. Miller used to claim that the indebtedness which Newfoundland incurred because of the railway and World War I was the *coup de grâce* to responsible government in 1933.

Newfoundland believed it was in its interest to remain a self-governing colony and in 1869 voted against joining the Dominion of Canada. But it rarely prospered. Dried fish did not fetch a large price, and there were swings in the price fish fetched abroad. At best it was a marginal economy. Government could be described as a merchant oligarchy. It had little impact in the outports except as a provider of largesse. Members elected to the legislature from the outport ridings were expected to champion the interests of their own constituents, to persuade government to channel public works programs in their direction and to remember them in patronage appointments. Such a system was not conducive to the development of local initiative or self-government, something which Miller used to deplore. The government seemed to have been aware of this gap and in 1890 enacted the creation of elected district boards responsible for public services; but since they had no authority to levy taxes and had to depend on government grants, they never grew into effective bodies. Consequently, and this was a point Miller would frequently harp on, unlike other parts of North America of those times, Newfoundlanders, instead of creating their own social service networks, looked to the government to provide them.

Natural disasters was an added feature of life in Newfoundland. Building stone was not available except on the west coast. Houses were built from wood since only the wealthy could afford brick or imported stone. As a consequence, towns were vulnerable to devastating fires. The worst was the Great Fire of 1892 which practically obliterated St. John's. Sensing that this was an opportunity to start a new venture, young Charles H. Miller, Leonard's father, and his future brother-in-law Elias Gittleson came to the city in 1897 from Halifax, Nova Scotia, and opened the US Picture and Portrait Company com-

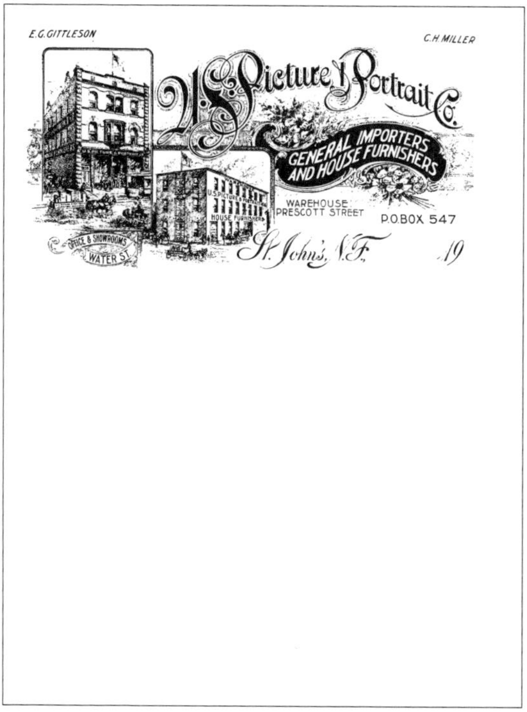

Letterhead – US Picture and Portrait Company
Courtesy Mrs. Yvette Brooks

monly known as the USP, a picture framing business which prospered and expanded into a flourishing house furnishings firm.

Like many Newfoundlanders, Miller was interested in genealogy. He was only too happy to rattle off his wife's ancestors but, strangely, never spoke about his own family nor did he leave anything in writing. His son Keith remembers visiting his uncle Bernard at the age of fourteen and noticing his cousins wearing yarmulkas; he assumed that since his father and uncle had been orphaned at an early age, his uncle had been raised by a Jewish family and had converted to their religion and that this accounted for the difference in religion! (Leonard married an Anglican and the children were raised Anglicans.) He reflected that it never crossed his mind that in fact his father had also been Jewish. He never questioned his father about his origins and only years later found out the truth. It was not that his father was ashamed of his race or practised concealment. He and his brother always remained on friendly terms and visited each other. It was just that he chose never to talk about his origins.* His brother was equally reticent about the family. Consequently, few details about Miller's forebears have survived. His father, Charles H. Miller, was born in 1876 in Germany, perhaps in Hamburg, one of a family of three boys and two girls. As a child he was taken by his parents to the U.S.A. and in 1890, according to a nephew, he became a naturalized American citizen at Portland, Maine. The family then moved to Halifax, Nova Scotia. In 1897 Charles came to St. John's with his future brother-in-law, Elias G. Gittleson, to start the USP company at 163-5 Water Street. Gittleson seems to have been the leading partner since in the St. John's City Directory for 1913 his name is listed ahead of Miller's with no rank while Miller is designated as Assistant Manager. Some years later Miller's brother, Michael, joined the firm as collector and Gittleson's brother Henry as secretary. In 1902 Charles Miller married his cousin Henrietta (Yetta) Miller in Port Chester, New York. Her parents came either from East or what was then called West Prussia. The Millers are described as heavy-set, speaking with a foreign accent and keeping to themselves. They and the Gittlesons occupied adjoining semi-detached houses at 72 and 74 LeMarchant Road. Three children were born to the Millers: Bernard in 1903 and Leonard in 1906. There was a girl who died in infancy.

* I did not come across any references to Miller's feelings concerning the deteriorating status of the Jews in Germany in the 1930s nor to any interventions on behalf of would be immigrants to Newfoundland.

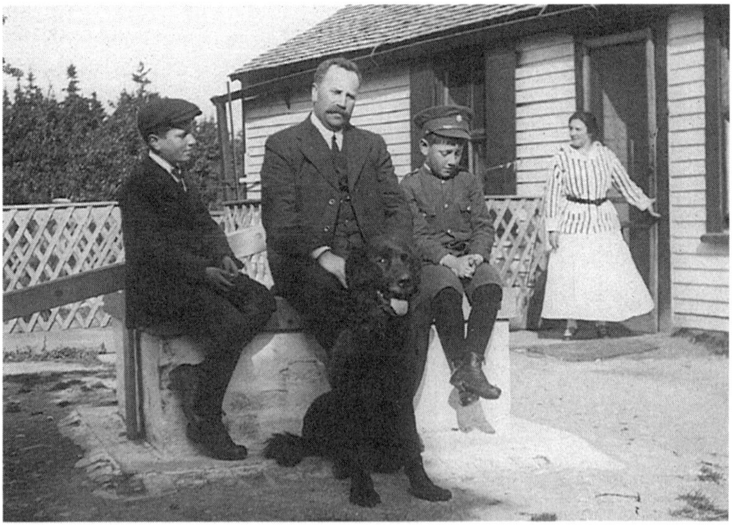

Rear view of "The Farm", Cornwall Avenue, St. John's. Charles Miller with Bernard (left) Leonard (right) Lizzie Miller at door. Courtesy Ms. Yvette Brooks

The Millers were comfortably off. Summers were spent at "The Farm," an extensive property close to St. John's from which, incidentally, it is said that Alcock and Brown took off on their transatlantic flight in 1919.

Unfortunately, a happy childhood ended in tragedy. One day in 1912, according to family tradition, the boys saw their mother being taken away so that she might "be made well again," but she never returned. She died while being operated on for an ectopic pregnancy. Their father's maiden sister, Lizzy, then came to help raise the boys.

In the winter of 1917-1918 several cousins from the U.S.A. came to visit the Millers and the Gittlesons in St. John's. Charles became engaged to one of them. The plan was for Charles and his American relatives to go as a group to New York for the wedding. But Minnie Gittleson, his sister, thought it would be improper for the engaged couple to travel together and persuaded Charles to follow separately on the next boat, the *Florizel*. But tragedy struck again. The *Florizel* was wrecked and Charles was one of those who perished. In Cassie Brown's gripping account of the disaster (replete with vignettes of a number of the passengers and crew) he appears only as a name in the list of those that drowned. It was said that Minnie felt herself responsible for her brother's death.

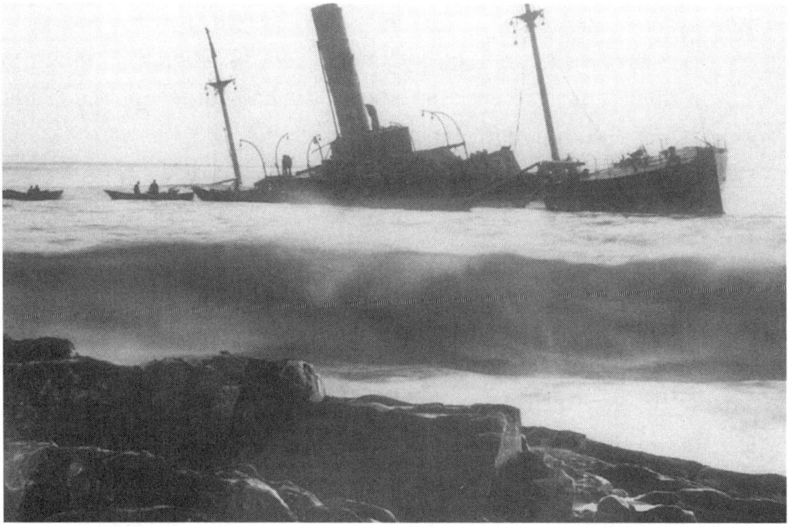

Wreck of SS Florizel, *Cappahayden, NF 23 February 1918 on which Leonard's father perished.* *Courtesy of Centre of Newfoundland Studies*

The Jewish community in St. John's in which the Miller boys grew up was always small.* Almost all had come from Russia fleeing the pogroms. Upon arrival they were desperately poor but like other Jewish communities there was a strong sense of responsibility to help new arrivals to get on their feet. Charles Miller, coming from a well established German-Jewish family in Halifax, ranked among the elite of St. John's Jewish society, "a cut above the others" in the words of a contemporary. To preserve its identity in such an alien environment was a constant battle for the society. The pressures and temptations to melt into the gentile world were great. To procure kosher meat was sometimes impossible for long periods and to observe the injunction against work on Saturdays was to suffer a financial penalty. There were more insidious pressures to assimilate. The children attended Protestant schools and were inevitably drawn into gentile society and many times ended marrying outside the faith. But perhaps the most decisive influence that encouraged assimilation was the rarity of "social" anti-semitism in Newfoundland. The vexatious discriminations and slurs to which Jews coming to the western world daily encountered, were frowned upon in Newfoundland in the days when they were still rife on the mainland. Dr. James McGrath, at one time Minister of Health, warned his daughter as she was going off to school in Montreal in the 1940s "not to return with strange [racist] ideas about the Jews." With the cards so stacked against them it was indeed a struggle for the Jews to maintain their identity. The more religious moved on to larger Jewish centres when their children reached their teens. Those who stayed on had to accept the likelihood of their children marrying gentiles.

Charles Miller was one of the founders of St. John's first Synagogue and his boys were raised as observant Jews. After their father was drowned, the sons were taken in by the Gittlesons next door. Aunt Minnie Gittleson was their father's sister. Bernard and Leonard attended the Methodist College. In those days two aims were uppermost in the minds of the parents or guardians of Jewish children: to see that they got the best possible education and that they stayed out of trouble with the law. It was widely feared that if a

* I am indebted to Alison Kahn's *Listen While I Tell You* for much that I have to say about the Jewish community in St. John's. For the sorry record of Newfoundland in not providing a haven for Jewish refugees in the 1930s (especially for much needed physicians), see Gerhard Bassler – *Sanctuary Denied.*

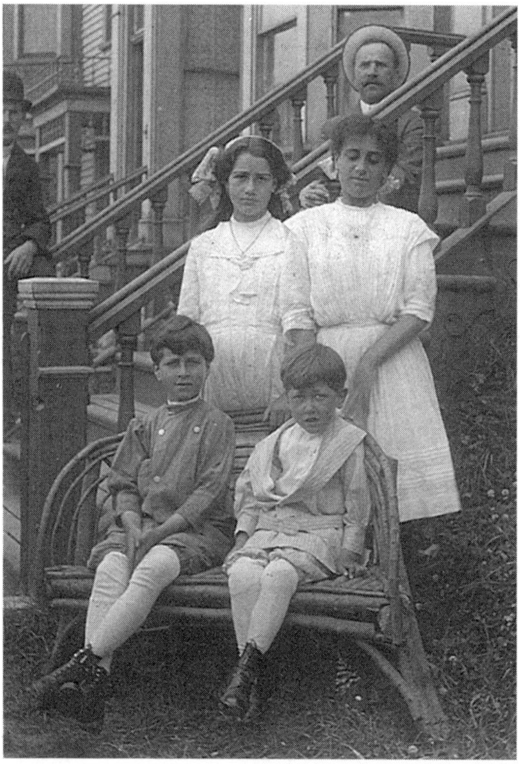

Family Group Seated: left to right Bernard, Leonard
Standing: Gittleson cousins, Charles seated on steps.
Courtesy Ms. Yvette Brooks

Jewish youth fell foul of the law "they would throw the book at you". The Miller boys managed to achieve both parental aims.

A Gittleson cousin remembers the youthful Leonard as "fair and more independent than Bernard; he was very nice to small children. At school he mingled and played with his schoolmates. He was well able to hold his own, but was not athletic". The Miller and Gittleson boys were given violin lessons, but met with "minimal success". Leonard's vocal skills were equally mediocre. Later when he used to attend church and sing hymns, his wife would be obliged to raise her voice to drown him out. When he became Deputy Minister he would observe the New Year's Day custom of St. John's society by dressing up in a morning coat, top hat and spats and, with his friends, doing the rounds of the various levees. Perhaps because 'good cheer' was offered at some of these places, he and his companions would arrive home happy and singing. That evening the

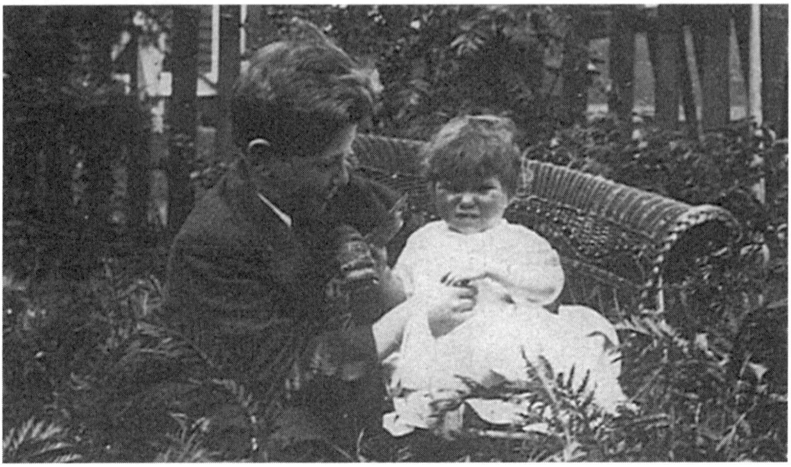

He loved children even then. Leonard and his cousin Yvette Gittleson circa 1918. Courtesy Mrs. Yvette Brooks.

Millers would throw their annual New Year's Day party and by the end of the evening Miller would have become sufficiently uninhibited to regale his guests with songs, sung not too tunefully. His favourites were "Prisoner's Son" and "Come, Come I Love You Only." This was the only day of the year the public saw Miller with his guard down.

What were Miller's hobbies if he had no "artistic talents"? At one time he must have known enough German to understand lectures during his stay in Vienna. In his spare time he enjoyed reading, particularly history with a special interest in Newfoundland. Like so many of his contemporaries, card games were where he relaxed. He was a competent bridge and poker player, but never for high stakes. The weekly poker games with his cronies were famous in their day. For a number of years he was an active member of the Kinsmen's Club and was a keen Mason rising to the position of Master of his Lodge. In a crowd Miller did not stand out one way or the other, a quality that was to stand him in good stead as a civil servant. His was a personality that did not invite or attract attention.

Profits from the USP were sufficient to pay for the Miller boys' university careers. Bernard went to McGill University, in Montreal, and after graduating with a Bachelor of Commerce degree settled in Trenton, New Jersey, where he married within his faith and worked as an accountant. He and his brother shared at least one trait: each was highly respected in his community. Leonard attended Dalhousie University, Halifax, Nova Scotia, graduating with a B.A. in 1926 and M.D. in 1930. During his summer vacations he worked at Connor's Drug Store in St. John's compounding and dispensing medications. This was to be his introduction to medicine.

He does not appear to have been an outstanding student, scoring an average of 56.9 percent in the first year and 62 percent in the final year. He did not fail any course but had only one Distinction, in physiology. He was a talented debater and was a zealous member of the university debating society. He also threw himself into student politics and at one time served as President of the Student Union. He particularly relished challenging a speaker on a point of order. So much power did he come to hold that it was said it was hopeless to run for the Student Council without his approval. Miller was not afraid to challenge authority. One professor was notorious for locking the door of the lecture room as the bell was still ringing. One day while the bell was ringing Miller began banging on the locked door. The irate professor opened the door and told Miller that he was late and began to shut the door again. Miller stopped him by putting his foot in and reminded him that the bell was still ringing and threatened to complain to the authorities if this happened again. It never did.

One thing was a shock to Miller. For the first time he encountered virulent anti-semitism. During his internship one staffman said to him ,"I don't want a Jew on my team."

After interning at the Victoria General Hospital, Halifax, Miller returned to St. John's in 1930 to start a private practice. Why he chose St. John's is a mystery. By this time he did not have a single relative there and Newfoundland was in the depths of the Great Depression and worse off than any other part of North America. The government was facing bankruptcy. But Miller loved Newfoundland and felt a tremendous loyalty towards his birthplace; perhaps this guided his return in such inauspicious times.

CHAPTER 3

Last Days of Responsible Government 1930 - 1934

The reason for Newfoundland's disastrous state in 1930 goes back to World War I which had saddled the country with heavy debts and the obligation to pay pensions to disabled veterans. Then in 1923 the government took over the bankrupt railway and its debts, but was never able to turn it into a profitable enterprise. Efforts to modernize the offshore fishing industry and to make it more competitive had foundered on the rocks of the innate conservatism of merchants and fishermen. The depressed state of fishing markets in the post-war years added to the misery of the outports. Successive governments showed little capacity for coping with the deteriorating finances. Reckless loans and deficit budgeting accelerated the descent into the financial abyss. By 1927, 40% of revenue was going into paying interest on the country's debt. The Depression administered the final blow to this rickety financial structure.

There was now the real danger of the government's defaulting on the interest on its bonds, something the Imperial government said it would not tolerate. Discussions were held between the UK, Canada and Newfoundland. Anglo-Canadian loans to meet the immediate financial needs were arranged. But it was widely realized that more long-term remedies were required to extricate the country from its financial quagmire. Scapegoats were sought for the unhappy state of affairs. A very obvious candidate was the system of government, made up by a coalition of interest groups, each vying for its

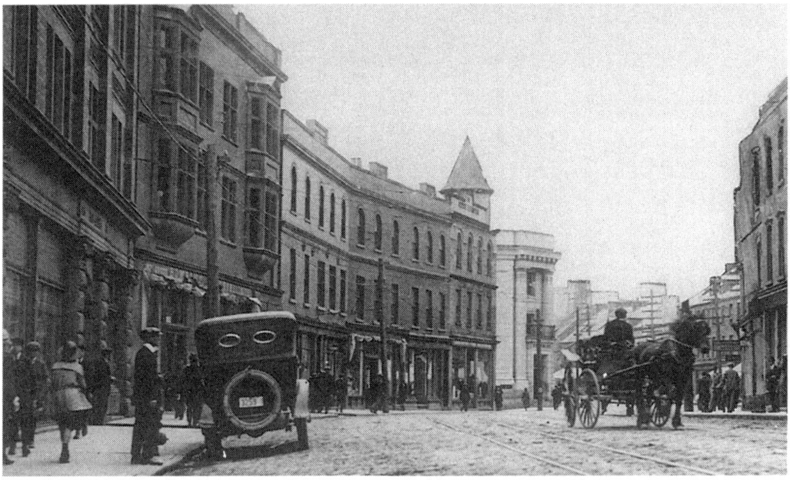

Water Street, St. John's circa 1925
Courtesy Provincial Archives of Newfoundland and Labrador

share of patronage and public works. What was needed, so it was argued, was "a rest from politics" and government by business-minded men to rescue the island's economy. This could only come about through abandoning self-government and replacing it by direct rule from the United Kingdom. This platform was championed by Frederick Alderdice and won him the 1932 election. The Imperial government responded by appointing a Royal Commission under the chairmanship of Lord Amulree to conduct an inquiry into the affairs of the Dominion and to make recommendations.[1] The Commission recommended "a Commission of Government" with full executive and legislative authority, appointed by and responsible to the UK government. Of practical significance: the Imperial Government should assume oversight of Newfoundland finances. The Amulree recommendations were accepted by the Newfoundland legislature and the Imperial government petitioned to implement them. Westminster responded with the Newfoundland Act of 1933 which came into force 16 February 1934, ending self-government.

The Royal Commission on Health and Public Charities, 1930 [2]

At this point it is necessary to turn to an action of the Newfoundland government in its closing days, one which was to have far-reaching consequences for the medical services of the island in the years to come. In 1930, perhaps at the prodding of the NMA, a Royal Commission on Health and Public Charities was appointed. Dr. H.M. Mosdell (1883 - 1944), of whom more will be heard later, was named secretary of the Commission. He had had a colourful career, starting life as a journalist before becoming a physician, which he forsook to return to journalism, and later entered politics and reached cabinet rank. Even after he stopped practice he maintained a keen interest in public health and seems to have been well-informed and abreast of developments in this field.

The findings and recommendations of the Commission were to shape health policy for the next few decades.[2] The Commissioners claimed that per capita expenditure on health and welfare compared favourably with Canada and USA but the reasons for the dismal results were inefficiency, unauthorized expenditure, duplication and divided authority. The cure lay in centralization and strict government control of all government-owned and operated health institutions and programs, a philosophy that was to dominate government health department policy for the next few decades and to influence Miller's thinking on health matters. The commissioners recommended a bureau of health and public welfare consisting of all the members of the Executive Council plus the Secretary of Health and Public Welfare under the chairmanship of the Colonial Secretary of Newfoundland.

They also recommended that the construction and maintenance of health facilities should remain under the Department of Public Works. This recommendation was to have unfortunate repercussions in the Smallwood era, leading to the construction of new hospitals and renovations in a haphazarded manner, without any regard to financial considerations or long-term planning. It was also to open the door to the exercise of patronage. The separation of the operation of health care from its buildings was to be a thorn in the side of Miller as Deputy Minister. Once a hospital was built the Department of Health was saddled with the cost of its equipment and salaries for the staff. Another recommendation was the creation of Medical Health Officers (MHO), salaried physicians responsible for public health programs and the treatment of indigents. It was as MHO that Miller was to start his career as a government official.

Children's health and the prevention of illness was prominent in the minds of the Commissioners. This required a survey before child health clinics could be established. The Commissioners also recommended that the government take over the district nursing services from The Newfoundland Outport Nursing and Industrial Association (NONIA). But the most memorable of the proposals of the Royal Commission was the one recommending a network of Cottage Hospitals on the model of those in the Scottish Highlands. (The Commission made no reference to the several Cottage Hospitals already in existence in the Dominion). Before its demise, the government enacted only those recommendations that were of an administrative and regulatory nature, including the establishment of a department of health and public welfare.[3]

Health Services 1924-1930

The medical scene in St. John's to which Miller returned in 1930 would not have been considered up to date. The population of the Dominion was about 289,588* and was serviced by 83 physicians.[1] St. John's with a population of about 39,886* had 23 physicians. There were no specialists; operations were still performed in homes. The largest institution (165 beds) was the government-owned General Hospital.[4] This was where the poor were treated. The government also operated the Hospital for Mental and Nervous Diseases now known as The Waterford Hospital (600 beds), the Sanatorium (250 beds) and the Home for the Infirm. For those who could pay there were two private hospitals, St.Clare's Mercy Hospital (50 beds) and the Grace General Hospital (50 beds), run by the Sisters of Mercy and the Salvation Army respectively.[4] Outside St. John's there were four small non-government hospitals: Corner Brook, Twillingate, Grand Falls and Grand Bank. A few solo physicians were scattered throughout the outports.

Paradoxically, the health services for more than half the colony were provided from abroad. The International Grenfell Association (IGA), a non-denominational social services mission founded to take care of the migratory fishing fleets to Labrador, had extended its services to the coastal communities of Labrador and the tip of the Northern Peninsula. It was supported entirely by charity, apart from a small annual subsidy from the Government. Successive governments were only too glad to leave it undisturbed.

* Census of Newfoundland and Labrador 1935 (The First Since 1921)

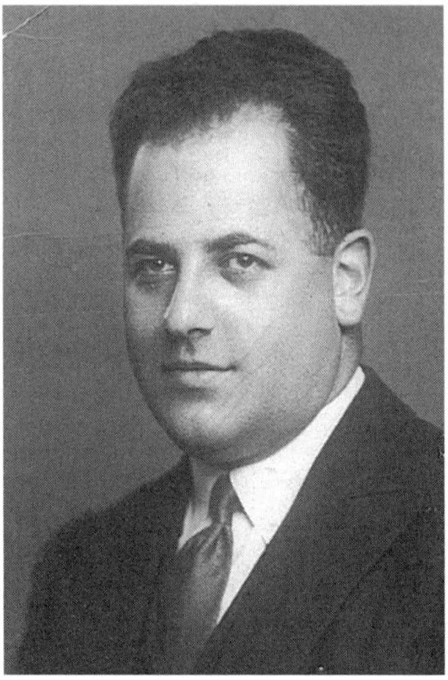

Leonard as a young man
Courtesy Mrs. L. Balderson

Practice In St. John's 1930-34

On returning to St. John's, Miller opened an office on Duckworth Street. His living quarters were on the floor above. He was a General Practitioner. This appears to have been a second choice; he would have preferred to be a pediatrician but he could not have supported himself as a consultant. Much of his work involved home visits and home deliveries, mainly on indigents. In the written memoir he left, Miller paints a grim picture of practice in St. John's in those times.[5] What struck him about some of the homes he visited was "the disappearance of household furniture. . . There was nothing in which one could wash one's hands." On one visit, to check a new born baby, Miller found the mother in tears because the midwife had taken her sewing machine since she had not been able to pay for her delivery. On another occasion, refusing to issue a death certificate until an autopsy could be performed on a dead baby, Miller was accused of keeping the baby above ground until his fee was paid. Physicians were hardly better off than their patients and Miller must have struggled to make ends meet. He tells of one physician who collected only two hundred and twenty-five dollars in six months of the thousands he had billed. He must have been relieved when in the autumn of 1930 he was asked to go as doctor on the Labrador boat sent to bring home migratory Newfoundland fishermen each year. It was also, he wrote, his first introduction to political pressure. On its return voyage the ship was carrying two patients, a boy dying from meningitis and a man less gravely ill, but with influential connections. Miller told the Captain that the first call should be the boy's home port. However, political pressures were brought to bear on the captain to discharge his more important passenger first. Miller stood firm and insisted on getting the boy home as quickly as possible, which was just as well since he died the day after reaching home. When it came to commenting on this incident years later, Miller, in his usual laconic way of referring to conduct of which he did not approve but which he had to tolerate, said, "This was my first experience with officialdom and the various aspects of it that I learned much about in later years." [5]

In June 1932 he began his government service as a part-time MHO in St. John's. The young physician was popular and was described as quite a party man, enjoying carousing with his friends. On one occasion he is said to have been responsible for smashing up a car. He maintained at least social links with the Jewish community; a lady remembers him as a frequent dinner guest at her parents' home.

One house call was to have a momentous impact on Miller's life. One evening, he writes, he was called by the mid-wife to take over a prolonged labour at Torbay, a small community several miles north of St. John's reached by a bumpy dirt road. Bad weather (it was snowing) added to the discomfort of the trip. The delivery was difficult and slow and lasted all night ending unfortunately in a grossly deformed baby that did not live. By this time it was dawn and Miller and the nurse prepared to return to St. John's. Just then a message arrived from the local Anglican clergyman (later Bishop John Meadon) inviting them to breakfast at the Rectory. "We willingly did and found that the clergyman's wife was confined to bed with laryngitis, but her sister was up and presided at breakfast. This was the lady I married the following year and we often laughed over the fact when the husband of the patient used to come and see me and remind me that if it hadn't been for him I wouldn't have met my wife."[5] Leonard Miller and Myra Chafe were married in September 1933 at Brigus. It was a social event attended by the elite.

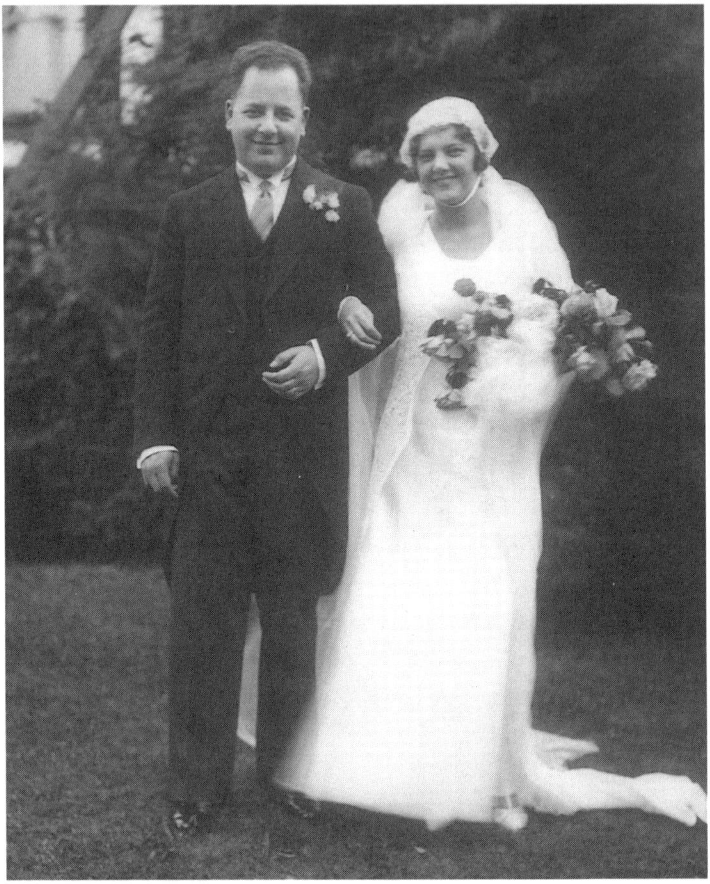

Wedding: Leonard and Myra (Chafe), Brigus, 11 September 1933
Courtesy Mrs. Lorraine Balderson

For their honeymoon the Millers went to Vienna for six months so that Leonard could pursue his interest in pediatrics. It was to be a most happy and unclouded union, bringing out a relaxed, playful side of the usually quiet, reserved Leonard. When he was away he would send Myra letters in "baby talk". With her he was able to let his hair down.

Never were angry voices heard in the Miller household. She was totally dependent on him and never wrote a cheque until after his death. She saw her task was to be at his side when needed and to devote her time to giving him a comfortable, happy home where he could relax after a stressful day at the office. Two children were born to the Millers, a daughter Lorraine (Balderson) and a son Keith.

At first the family lived on Duckworth Street, but during the war he had their ideal home built on Forest Road, "a home for Myra" as he was wont to say. In their early married life the Millers were able to afford a cook and a maid. Perhaps because of his own parentless youth Miller took care to give time to his children. He was always around for meals even if it meant going back to the office in the evening. He never pushed them and is described by his daughter "a whole bundle of love." Miller was not athletic; his only exercise was walking back and forth to his office.* While his son cannot recall playing catch with his father in the backyard, he remembers frequent fishing or trouting trips, as they are called in Newfoundland. Miller was not a handyman around the house. He did the chores and mowed the lawn but that was the extent of his usefulness. Keith remembers his father trying to figure out how to operate a stirrup pump fire extinguisher (a mandatory piece of equipment in every house during the war) and hoping that an occasion for its use would never arise.

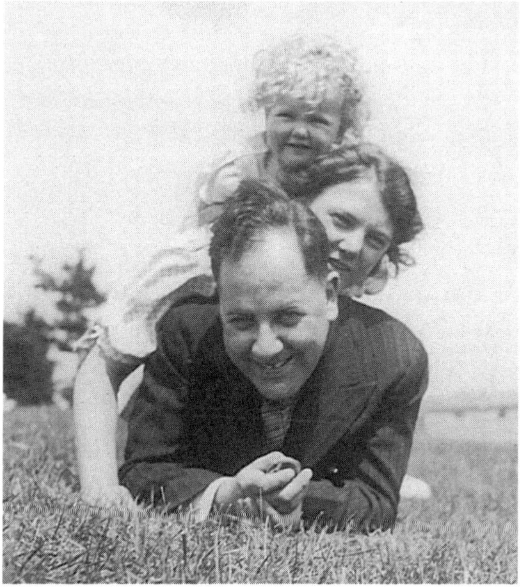

Leonard relaxing with Myra and Lorraine
Courtesy Mrs. Lorraine Balderson

* This cannot have been a strenuous form of activity. During Miller's career, the Department of Health was housed successively in the old museum building, Duckworth Street and then in a temporary war-time building, Fort William (just behind Miller's home), before moving much further out to the Confederation Building in 1959, presumably ending the daily walks.

A quirk of Miller's was his fondness for the nearby fire station . Nothing seemed to give him greater pleasure than to take his children, and later the grandchildren, up to the station, sit them on the trucks and try out whatever equipment the firemen would let them tackle. He was on first name terms with them and was a much loved figure at the station.

His approval meant much to his children and grandchildren. One grandson had reached a stage in life when he was drifting and going nowhere. His grandfather sat him down and in so many words told him that it was a shame to see a young man with obvious talents going to waste. This devastating *exposé* was like a bombshell to the young man and he described his reaction: "It was the only time I heard him raise his voice to me and even then he wasn't shouting. It made a tremendous impact on me. It made me stop in my tracks and reevaluate where I was going. It was the turning point of my life. I can never be too thankful to him for turning me around. It was then that I decided to become a doctor like him and in the same field, preventive medicine."

One incident stands out in his son's memory since it showed his father's sensitivity to the feelings of others. Keith, his wife and Leonard were about to embark on a ferry. Suddenly the wife exclaimed that she had left her rings in the ladies room. To avoid hurt feelings and embarassment, turning to Keith, Leonard said *sotto voce*, "Keep your mouth shut."

Before marriage Miller appears to have been a thoroughly assimilated Jew. Inevitably, marriage to a devoted Anglican like Myra loosened whatever moorings remained to tie him to Judaism. He continued to have friendly but somewhat formal relations with members of the Jewish community. Still, childhood associations are not easily forgotten. He bequeathed his Prayer Shawl and Prayer Book to an old Jewish friend, Maurice Wilansky. When they were growing up Miller's children remembered him as an occasional attendant at St. Thomas's Church (his wife's church). Years later he was confirmed in the Anglican Church and became a regular attendant, although he admitted to the clergymen who received him into the Church to certain doctrinal reservations . The nature of these reservations has not been disclosed but they do not appear to have been a barrier to his reception. Ever afterwards he was an active attendant at St. Thomas's. The high regard he was held in is shown in the tribute to him in the church bulletin on the occasion of his retirement as "one of our most faithful parishioners" and as one whose career had been "tempered by justice, mercy and understanding for people in their illness and need."

In such a private and reticent person as Miller his innermost beliefs can only be surmised. From conversations with him I was left with the impression that his religion was not something to be paraded. Certainly his strict code of conduct extended into every facet of his life. He once expressed his disapproval to me of a married doctor for bringing his mistress to the annual banquet of the NMA. In the days of his "youthful zeal," as he describes them, he seemed to have felt that it was his duty to rebuke those who erred.[5] Once when he was conducting a home delivery, finding that the parents of the baby were not married, "[I told the father] in the plainest words that I could find, that he could not continue bringing bastards into the world. I shall never forget his reply. He looked me straight in the eye and said, 'Doctor, there are a lot of good people in this town who are bastards.' [5]

Chapter 3 – Notes

1. CNS Newfoundland Royal Commission 1933. HM Stationery Office, Adastral House, Kingsway London, WC2.

2. CNS Newfoundland Royal Commission on Health and Public Charities, First Interim Report. St. John's, King's Printer, 1930.

3. PANL An Act Respecting Health and Public Welfare. Acts of the General Assembly of Newfoundland. 1931.

4. WDPC Vanderlehr R.A. Heering R.E. Report of a Survey on Civil Health Services As They Relate to the Health of Armed Forces in Newfoundland. United States Public Health Service 3 December 1940. Unpublished.

5. NRC Miller, L.A. Memoir, unpublished.

CHAPTER 4

Commission of Government 1934 - 1944

History 1934 - 44

Commission of Government was inaugurated in February 1934. It reduced Newfoundland to the status of being little more than a colony of the UK, although to spare Newfoundlanders' feelings it was attached to the Dominions' Office. Full executive and legislative authority, subject to approval by Westminster, was vested in six commissioners nominated by the Secretary of State for Dominion Affairs. Each Commissioner was in charge of a department. Three were to come from the UK and three from Newfoundland. The Governor chaired the Commission and held the deciding vote. One of the first tasks of the new government was to rename and reorganize the ministries of the days of Responsible Government to reflect Newfoundland's change in status and the new regime's political leanings.[1]

The old department of Health and Public Welfare was renamed the department of Public Health and Welfare (PH&W) and placed under a commissioner. The chief civil servant in the new department was given the title of secretary for PH&W. What were considered the three most important departments, Finance, Natural Resources and Public Utilities, were reserved for the UK commissioners. PH&W did not rank among these and was left under a

Newfoundlander. Commission of Government has hardly enjoyed a good word from contemporaries or later. It has been accused of being paternalistic and secretive and failing to train Newfoundlanders in self government.

But the change in regime produced some easing of Newfoundland's financial burdens. The Imperial Government met the shortfall in interest payments on Newfoundland bonds and Newfoundland now qualified for loans under the Colonial Development Fund. However, efforts to turn around the economy by modernizing the antiquated fishing industry and land settlement came to nought. What did bring better times was the outbreak of World War II. St. John's now became a major gathering point for convoys crossing the Atlantic, and Gander the hopping-off point for the Ferry Command of the Allied Air Forces. These activities required military installations and airports and accommodation for those operating them. Undreamt of opportunities for employment now materialized. The improved standard of living also benefited the health of the population.

The one department of the Commission of Government which has received unstinted praise was PH&W[2] The Commissioner was Mr. (later Sir) John C. Puddester (1881-1947)* and under him as secretary for PH&W, Dr. H.M. Mosdell. Miller was enthusiastic in his praise of both of these men. "I believe that more was accomplished [during their tenure] than has been accomplished since."[3] Both had been prominent politicians in the days of Responsible Government, the very regime which was supposed to be responsible for the country's deplorable state. Although they had been in opposing parties they managed to work together reasonably harmoniously, but more importantly they complemented each other. One reason for their success was that, unlike the UK commissioners, they were familiar with the local scene and knew what might work and what wouldn't. Another was that Mosdell had been secretary of the Royal Commission of 1930. He was able to persuade Puddester, and through him the other commissioners, that, strapped as they were for funds, expenditures on health were imperative.

It was in the field of preventive medicine that the government could hope to have highest return on its expenditure. With almost

* He was knighted in 1939 when King George VI visited Newfoundland

30% of the adult population on the dole, malnutrition was assuming almost epidemic proportion. Malnutrition had perhaps always been present and probably was one of the causes for the poor physical fitness of so large a proportion of the population. In World War I, 47% of the volunteers and 57% of conscripts were rejected on medical grounds,[4] and in World War II, during the building boom of the American bases, labour had to be imported from the mainland, because so many Newfoundland applicants were rejected for health reasons.[5]

The malnutrition encountered in Newfoundland was due to a deficiency of vitamins and minerals and not calories. For this reason it had attracted the notice of nutritionists interested in documenting the clinical effects of deficiencies in vitamins and essential minerals. The government addressed the problem of beriberi by distributing whole wheat bread to those on the dole, but the experiment met with so much resistence that in 1944 the government accepted the advice of the the Nutritional Council of the NMA to allow the importation of only Vitamin B and iron-enriched flour. At the same time, the Nutritional Council recommended a nutritional survey of the province. The Commissioner of PH&W accepted this advice and the survey documented deficiency of vitamins A, C and riboflavin, although there was adequate intake of calories, protein and fat. Dietary calcium content was low.[5]

The investigators also made a number of recommendations to the Commissioner, separate from their report, the most important being Vitamin A fortification of margarine, nutritional education and free milk for school children. Miller, by this time Director of Medical Services, agreed with the picture the investigators painted and supported their recommendations. In 1947 free milk was given to school children and calcium was required to be added to flour and Vitamin A to margarine putting Newfoundland in the forefront of enlightened dietary legislation. Miller had one reservation about the Adamson survey: it described those examined as "somewhat slow in mental reactions and lacking in initiative. This was especially noticeable in the behaviour of their children. They were apathetic and abnormally subdued."[5] He warned that such words would provoke an outcry on the island and advised the team to express the same idea in terms less apt to give offence. His advice was ignored, and what he had predicted occurred. A repeat survey in 1947 showed marked improvements in intake of vitamins A, B and riboflavin, but not Vitamin C.[6] With increased prosperity after Confederation, vitamin deficiencies disappeared.

What part did Miller have in the enlightened nutritional measures of the government? He was president of the NMA in 1943 when the resolution recommending Vitamin B-enriched flour was passed, but nothing in writing has survived to indicate how active he was in pushing for better nutritional practices.

Another public health interest was tuberculosis. Newfoundland had the highest rate in North America and it was the leading cause of death until 1947. The magnitude of its impact can be grasped by recalling that it killed more people in both world wars than enemy action.[7] Measures to curtail the disease had begun in the days of Responsible Government by a combination of government and voluntary initiatives. In 1908 the Newfoundland Association for the Prevention of Consumption, later to become the Newfoundland Tuberculosis Association (NTA) and finally the Newfoundland Lung Association, was founded with the aim of prevention through education, using teachers as the vehicle for reaching the public.[8] Then in 1916 a 52 bed sanatorium was opened in St. John's; but these were pitiful measures to direct against an epidemic of such magnitude. In fairness to the government, so short of funds, mass diagnostic surveys and treatment of the kind then being pioneered in Saskatchewan at no cost to the benficiaries, were out of the question.[9] The in-coming Commision of Government wisely decided to do nothing until it had taken stock of the situation. It then rapidly made up for lost time by adopting measures that had proved so successful elswhere[9]. With support from the Rockefeller Foundation it conducted a survey of the prevalence of tuberculosis in parts of the Avalon Peninsula. It expanded the sanatorium to 300 beds, started a vigorous public education program through the schools and by radio and commenced BCG vaccinations.[10] In 1937 the Avalon Health Unit was established with Dr. J. McGrath in charge for screening the population on the Avalon Peninsula, using a mobile van equipped with an X-Ray machine. Some time later the NTA purchased and equipped a vessel, renamed The Easter Seal, for conducting mass screening of the outports. While Miller took an interest in the anti-tuberculosis programs, he left the management in McGrath's capable hands. In 1946 McGrath was responsible for producing a film under the auspices of the NTA called *The Silent Menace*, a twenty minute excellent state-of-the-art movie on tuberculosis.[7] He was the narrator and Miller appears briefly applying patch tests but saying nothing.

Commission of Government was to confer lasting benefits in the training of a Civil Service after the Whitehall model. Its function was not to come up with bright revolutionary policies, but to see that things kept running no matter what storms might blow up in the political arena. Miller was a product of this school.

But in the health field, it was the commencement of a network of cottage hospitals for which Commission of Government is best remembered.

Professional Life 1934-1944

When the Millers came back from their honeymoon in 1934, the Commission of Government had just taken office. Miller was invited to become a full-time MHO at a salary of three thousand six hundred dollars per annum.[11] Because of his pediatric training he was given responsibility for antenatal and pediatric health programs in St. John's. The major health scourges he had to grapple with, malnutrition and contagious diseases, stemmed from poverty. Miller was now committed to a career in public health. He realized that he would have to pursue postgraduate studies in this field if his career was to advance. In 1935 he obtained a Rockefeller Foundation fellowship which enabled him to take a leave of absence for one year, go to Boston to study for a certificate in public health at Harvard University. Later (1939) he obtained a Master's Degree in Public Health (MPH), presumably by correspondence.

Upon his return Miller took up once again his duties as MHO. The workload kept increasing and he never took a holiday.[12] However, his name came before a wider audience when he became the Child Welfare Association nominee to the Commission of Enquiry on Housing and Town Planning, under the chairmanship of Mr. Justice (later Sir) Brian Dunfield.[13] The Commission confirmed what many already knew, that much of the housing in the poorer quarters was substandard, overcrowded, and without proper sanitary facilities, in no small measure the result of hasty rebuilding after the Great Fire of 1892. Dunfield, according to Miller, dominated the commission.[14] But presumably Miller wrote the chapter on housing and health which cited figures to show the connection between overcrowded substandard houses and disease.[13]

The Commission recommended a code of building regulations and the institution of a housing corporation, authorized to expropriate land on which to build low-cost housing. The Commission of Government adopted the recommendations but the implementation of the low-cost housing scheme ran into fierce opposition from landlords and their supporters threatened with expropriation. For his part, as a doctor and a pragmatist, Miller believed establishing the poor in newer housing developments would be useless without any increase in income.[15]

Three events stand out during the period Miller was MHO. They display different facets of his character.

The first concerned the Department of PH&W and the NMA. Relations between the two followed an uneven course. The department frequently solicited the advice of the NMA but was quick to resent what it considered to be unwarranted intrusions into its own bailiwick. On the other hand the NMA saw itself as the advocate of the doctors, particularly when it came to defending them from arbitrary treatment by the department. A clash occurred in 1938. The details are not clear but it seems that the department felt that the contracts it had with part-time MHOs were too loosely worded.[3] For example, the practice had developed of physicians charging extra fees for immunizations. The department decided that new contracts were needed, ones which were more precisely worded and which would make it clear that immunizations were included in the services covered by the contracts. Without consultation with the NMA, the department sent out the new contracts requiring the part-time MHOs signatures within three months upon pain of termination of service. The NMA executive committee (of which Miller was a member) examined the new contract and in a letter to its members drew their attention to clauses it considered detrimental to their interests. It is said the Executive Committee advised members not to sign the new contracts. In fact, eventually all the part-time MHOs signed, with one exception. Puddester and Mosdell took offence at what they regarded as an uncalled for meddling in a departmental matter.

The dispute put Miller in a difficult position, he was a full time MHO but also a member of the NMA executive. It is a credit to his skills that he came through the storm unscathed without incurring the ill will of either party, probably because in the NMA executive discussions on the tactics to be adopted he advised caution and avoided inflammatory comments.

In 1942 Miller became President of the NMA and with the conclusion of his term of office ceased to be actively involved in the affairs of the association. Henceforth he was to play a most useful part as a bridge between the government and the profession.

The next event shows Miller sticking to his guns. During the war the Department of PH&W had started a program of radio broadcasting aimed at teaching good health practices. Miller was responsible for preparing and giving these talks. He notified the Newfoundland Broadcasting Company of his intention of speaking on venereal diseases.[16] (He had given a talk on this subject before without stirring any controversy.) St. John's, like all war-time port cities, was plagued with sexually transmitted diseases (STD). The authorities were determined to alert the public to the magnitude and dangers of the epidemic. Miller was told by the secretary of the broadcasting company that the topic was prohibited on the airways. Miller felt so strongly about the need to educate the public on STD that he took his case to Sir John Puddester who took up the cudgels on his behalf, citing the example of the Archbishop of York who had just given a radio talk on STD on the BBC. All to no avail. Perhaps it was wishful thinking to assume that the example of an Anglican Archbishop would carry weight with the Roman Catholic secretary of a Newfoundland broadcasting company. The broadcasting company refused to lift its ban. Miller told Puddester that it would be intolerable to submit to lay censorship and recommended discontinuation of the talks. Puddester concurred.[16] Evidently things were eventually patched up and Miller resumed his talks a few years later.

It may seem surprising that at one time he was a well known broadcaster. As a speaker and lecturer, his voice was low and delivery slow, monotonous and somewhat boring, but in spite of these obvious disadvantages, the content could hold an audience's attention.

The third event shows Miller going to battle for his rights, canny enough not to act alone but to choose the occasion and the timing so that he was bound to win his case.

In the Spring of 1943, five key full-time salaried physicians, one of them Miller, presented a joint memorial to the Commissioner of PH&W, Sir John Puddester, requesting a 30% increase in salaries.[17] Mosdell wrote separately to the Commissioner supporting their request in principle. Dr. D. E. Bennett, Superintendent of the Hospital for Mental and Nervous Diseases, is said to have been the instigator behind this *démarche*. Each of the five presented a memorandum setting down his case for an increase in pay. Not surprisingly, each was characterized by a certain degree of special pleading, and in this respect Miller's did not differ from the others.[12] He listed the reasons which had led him to accept the invitation to join the department as a full-time MHO in 1934, a liking for public health and a belief that although the remuneration was low, as conditions improved so would the salary. The salary increase had not happened, but now he found himself overworked and making far less than he could in private practice. He submitted that "a medical man heading a subdivision of your department is entitled to a standard of living at least equal to that of the average private practitioner." He concluded by hinting that financial considerations might compel him to leave government service. This was not an entirely fair representation of his treatment by government. The Commissioner of Finance, to whom the memorial and memoranda had been sent, pointed out that each of the physicians (except Bennett) had periodically moved up the salary scale even during the war years. Furthermore, from his inquiries their salaries were not out of line with those for comparable posts in Canada and the UK. Finally, the Commissioner said, if the government were to capitulate to their demands how could it hope to hold the line with more junior staff for similar increases? He also used the well-worn excuse that there was a war on and it was unpatriotic to ask for a raise before it was over.[17]

After discussing the memorial with the Commissioner of Finance, Puddester came back to the MHOs with an offer which was declined. At this point there appears to have been a misunderstanding .

The Commissioner withdrew his offer, claiming that the five had added extra conditions. They on their part, accused him of abruptly withdrawing it because they had only sought clarification on a couple of points. A few weeks later four of the five sent a joint memorial to Puddester threatening to resign unless the government reopened negotiations.[18] Bennett refused to be party to this ultimatum and dissociated himself from this step of his colleagues. The government, faced with the possibility of losing four essential employees, had no choice but to reopen negotiations. Eventually an agreement was reached for a figure less than the 30% originally requested. The Commissioner of Finance in endorsing this agreement for transmission to the Secretary of State for Dominion Affairs for his approval, singled out Miller and J.E. Josephson (Chief Pathologist and Director of Medical Laboratories) as "especially good men whom it would be tragedy to lose through lack of opportunity."[17]

The incident illustrates the dilemma facing salaried employees in government-operated essential services who seek to better their work conditions. What kinds of pressure are justifiable? When it came to the bottom line the four acted no differently than other similarly situated employees, then and now. But perhaps the most surprising aspect was that of the five, it was Bennett, not Miller, who drew back from exerting what could be construed as improper pressure on the government.

In 1944 when Mosdell died, Puddester proposed replacing him by Lewis Crummey, a layman who was the assistant secretary for public health and welfare, while offering the positions of Chief Medical Officer and Assistant Medical Officer to Miller and McGrath respectively.[19] Presumably they would have been junior to Crummey. They must have protested, because while Crummey was appointed secretary of public health and welfare, Miller was advanced to the newly created position of Director of Medical Services and took over the medical duties that previously had been discharged by Mosdell.[20] His salary was raised from five thousand five hundred to six thousand dollars per annum.[20] McGrath was appointed Assistant Director of Medical Services. Where Crummey fitted into this administrative structure is not stated.

Chapter 4 – Notes

1. PANL An Act to Make Temporary Provision for the Management of the Public Service, 1934-02-17.

2. The St. John's Evening Telegram (editorial) 1944 02 02.

3. NRC Miller, L.A. Memoir. (Unpublished) .

4. Overton ,James. *Nutrition.* In *Twentieth Century Newfoundland's Explorations*, Edited by James Hiller and Peter Neary, Breakwater, St. John's, Newfoundland, AlC 6E6. 1994.

5. Adamson, J.D. et al *Medical Survey of Nutrition in Newfoundland*, Canadian Medical Association Journal 52 (3): 227-42 1945.

6. Cuthbertson, D.P. *Report on Nutrition in Newfoundland*, London H.M. Stationary Office 1947.

7. PANL *The Silent Menace* Lee Wulff Production 1946 (Movie).

8. House, Edgar *Light at Last. Triurnph and Tuberculosis in Newfoundland and Labrador.* St. John's Jesperson Press 1981.

9. Houston, C. Stuart *R.G. Ferguson. Crusader Against Tuberculosis.* Hannah Institute and Dundurn Press Toronto and Oxford 1991. p. 66-67, 72-84.

10. McGrath, J. *Newfoundland's Greatest Medical Problem.* Address to the St. John's Rotary Club. The St. John's Evening Telegram 1942-01-30.

11. PANL GN 38 S6-1- 1.

12. PANL GN38 S6-5-2 LAM to JCP 1943-04-01.

13. CNS Commission of Enquiry on Housing and Town Planning in St. John's. Third Interim Report (St. John's, 1943).

14. Lewis, J. Shrimpton, M. *Policy Making in Newfoundland During the 1940's: The Case of the St. John's Housing Corporation*, Canadian Historical Review 65 (2): 209-39 1984.

15. *One In Nine.* (Editorial) The St. John's Evening Telegram 1944-02-02.

16. PANL GN38 S6-5-2 LAM to JCP 1943-07-23, JCP to RSF 1943-07-29 LAM to JCP 1943-09-03.

17. PANL GN38 S6-5-2.

18. PANL GN38 S6-5-2 J McG, LAM, JEJ, and ESP to JCP 1943-07-27.

19. PANL GN 38/Sl-1 Minutes of Commission Government 602-44 1944-06-26.

20. PANL GN38/ S6-1-3 Memo JCP 1944-07-04.

CHAPTER 5

Director of Medical Services

When Miller became Director of Medical Services (DMS) technically he was the successor to Mosdell, but perhaps the new title underlined the point that his authority was not as extensive as his predecessor's. Welfare and the government-owned hospitals in St. John's were expressly excluded from his responsibilities.[1]

The reason for this limitation was not stated, but some years later the government health institutions in St. John's (but not welfare) were added to his responsibilities. Miller was now in the position to determine or at least influence policy. In fact the last five years of Commission of Government were to be years of maintaining and improving what had been laid down before the war. Quiet, unspectacular and efficient administration was the order of the day, not plunging into new ventures. There were solid achievements, including construction of a 220–bed sanatorium at Corner Brook and expansion of the General Hospital. Two Canadian Armed Forces hospitals in St. John's were turned over to the government which attached one to the sanatorium and the other, adjacent to the General, was turned into an orthopedic hospital.

Now that he was in the seat of authority, Miller could bring his own ideas and goals to bear on health policy. Two speeches he gave during this decade showed the direction of his thoughts. The first was entitled *A Plea for Public Health.*[2] Miller had been trained in public health which in those days encompassed sanitation, control of communicable diseases and health protection and education. He advocated these approaches as the most cost-effective for raising levels of health in Newfoundland. No one could quarrel with these sentiments, then or now. It was not that Miller discounted the need for more hospital beds and the most up-to-date equipment and facilities for the treatment of the acutely ill, but that throughout his career his guiding philosophy was that treatment and preventive programs must proceed in parallel by establishing priorities and long-term planning. Unlike many who blow the trumpet for preventive medicine, Miller, having been a general practitioner for several years before choosing a career in preventive medicine, knew that treatment and prevention were not alternatives but were complementary to each other. His views carried weight because of his first-hand experience in both fields.

An issue that Miller believed would be coming to the fore after the war was health insurance for the entire population. This was the subject of his presidential address to the NMA in 1943.[3] He noted that people were beginning to accept the idea that the state did have a stake in the patient-physician relationship. The major part of his address was a summary of recent discussions on health insurance in the Canadian House of Commons and the Canadian Medical Association (CMA). The latter had come out in favour of "The Principal of Health Insurance." Miller then summarized the situation in Newfoundland, noting that part of the population was already covered by government operated services but the people for whom assistance really was necessary, were those "of moderate means" who could be bankrupted by medical costs. After citing a number of case histories with this outcome, Miller concluded by saying, "I think you will agree that state intervention is necessary in such cases." Miller did not pretend to have the answer to what form this should take. His thinking seems to have been the same as that advocated twenty years later by the CMA, that government intervention was required only on behalf of those who could not afford to insure themselves. He concluded by calling on the NMA to collect data and "to help in finding a solution to the problem of securing adequate medical care for . . . Newfoundlanders." In other words it was the responsibility of the medical association to be pro-active and come up with the answers.

In 1947 Sir John Puddester died. The new Commissioner for PH & W, Herman Quinton, was from all accounts a less forceful personality, which left Miller free to run the department as he saw fit. The last four years of the Commission of Government were an interregnum. The Attlee Government in the UK was anxious to divest itself of burdens of which it viewed Newfoundland as one. Shortly after the end of the war a national convention was elected to advise the Imperial authorities on the future government of the country. The convention constituted a committee to report on health and welfare of the island. It reported that by measures of a nation's health such as infant mortality and tuberculosis rates, Newfoundland was far behind Canada and the USA.[4] (It is apparent the achievements in health under the Commission of Government had only been relative compared to previous regimes in Newfoundland and not to the standards of other countries.)

Early on the Imperial authorities had made it clear that if Newfoundland chose to return to responsible government, it would not receive any financial assistance from the UK government should it get into financial difficulties. It was apparent to any farsighted person that the relative prosperity of the fishing industry could not last, and that the only practical solution for Newfoundland's unpredictable financial state was union with Canada. When the country voted to join Canada, on 22 July 1948, Miller began to plan for the future.

Chapter 5 – Notes

1. PANL GN 38 S6-1-3 Memo JCP 1944-07-04. GN54, GN26.

2. Miller, L.A. *A Plea For Public Health*, Nova Scotia Medical Bull. 21: 346-50 1942.

3. ANLMA Miller, L.A. *The People, The Doctor and The State*, Presidential Address to the NMA 1943. Unpublished

4. CNS FF 1033 .5 N55 Newfoundland National Convention 1946-48. Reports of Committees; Vol. 3 Health and Welfare 1948.

CHAPTER 6

Deputy Minister and National Health Grants

On the 1st of April 1949 Newfoundland became Canada's tenth province. Shortly afterwards an election was held and the Liberal party under the leadership of J.R. Smallwood was swept into power. Smallwood was to remain Premier without a break for over 22 years and during that period came to exercise almost absolute powers. With the end of Commission of Government all civil service positions legally lapsed. The new government started with a clean slate, free to hire whom it wished. The old Department of PH & W was split into two, Health and Public Welfare, with H.W. Quinton the last Commissioner of PH & W staying on in charge of health with the new title of Minister of Health. A few months later he was replaced by J.R. Chalker. Shortly after his appointment he recalls a visit from Miller, who asked to be considered for the position of Deputy Minister of Health. Chalker had known Miller for a number of years and his reputation. "In the days of Commission of Government, Miller had come to be regarded as the authority on the administration of all Health matters. I certainly thought him the ideal candidate for the post and suggested so to Smallwood. Smallwood told me that in Canada it was the prerogative of Provincial Premiers not Ministers of departments to appoint Deputy Ministers. I was disappointed. Smallwood, I knew had someone else in mind for the position. But shortly afterwards he did appoint Miller to the position of Deputy Minister." Smallwood was later to tell Chalker, "I didn't appoint Miller at your suggestion, but at the recommendation of Paul Martin, The Federal Minister of National Health and Welfare (NH&W)".

Soon afterwards, Chalker visited Ottawa and was told by Martin: "Mr. Chalker you are a very lucky man to have Miller as your Deputy Minister and so is Canada." So far had Miller's reputation already travelled.

Confederation brought the extension of Canada's social network to the new province. This had a major impact on the outports where family allowances and increased old age pensions for the first time put large amounts of cash into the people's pockets, leading to the end of the old 'barter truck' system. From the point of view of health services the most worthwhile benefit was Newfoundland's qualifying for funding of projects under the Federal National Health Grants Program (NHGP) which had been instituted in 1945. Its purpose was to "assist the provinces in the development, improvement and extension of their health services and to promote a working partnership between the Dominion and the Provinces in the field of health."[1] A sum was allocated for use by each province annually, computed on a basic grant and the size of its population. The terms of the NHGP were so broad that almost any health project qualified for support.

Miller was well aware of the key role that funds from this source would play in improving health services, and in the months before and just after Confederation he began to prepare the groundwork for tapping them. Firstly, he wrote the NMA asking for suggestions for projects for which funding could be applied.[2] Secondly, he recommended to the Commissioner of PH&W the appointment of a health planning committee. The Commissioner acted on this suggestion. Meanwhile, he had started a correspondence with Dr. F.W. Jackson, Director of the NHGP, requesting information on the guidelines projects must meet to qualify for acceptance. Jackson provided a list of projects which had recently been approved by the Minister of NH & W and suggested that before any application was forwarded to the Minister it should first be sent to him for vetting to see if it met the guidelines.[3] Miller accepted the offer and over the next few years sent him a number of projects covering almost every aspect of health care for preliminary screening.

Soon after Confederation, Jackson visited Newfoundland and over the years a warm friendship and an extensive correspondence arose between the two men. But it took several years before it reached the 'Dear Fred' and 'Dear Len' stage. In the early years of union with Canada, Miller sought to use this source of money to its limit. Indeed, Newfoundland's utilization of its share of the NHGP exceeded that of any other province.[4] Looking back from 1956, Miller listed what he believed had been the twelve most important ongoing completed projects.[5] They covered a wide range and included, amongst other items, training of personnel, purchase of diagnostic equipment, salary for an internist (I. Rusted), provision of BCG vaccine, construction of several cottage hospitals, the setting up of nursing stations and the creation of a planning section for "providing information and services rendered unavailable and those still needed." Obviously, even then Miller appreciated the need for long term planning.

The friendship between the two blossomed beyond their involvement in the grants program, and Miller began to seek Jackson's assistance in other matters. When the iron ore mines in Western Labrador were in the planning stage in 1950 it became imperative to plan the townsite that would grow up around the mines. In response to a request from Miller, Jackson sent him the blueprints of a recently built mining town.[6]

Jackson had a high regard for Miller. In acknowledging receipt of a health promotion brochure, Jackson complemented Miller on its quality and requested more copies for distribution to other provincial departments of health. The close friendship between Jackson and Miller shows the high reputation that Miller enjoyed in Ottawa at the time of Confederation. Throughout his career Miller had his frustrations, and his son has the impression that in the 1950s he seriously considered job opportunities with the federal government.

The NHGP continued until medicare came into being. Indeed, Miller stated that from the beginning, the philosophy behind the grants was that they were "a step necessary to help provide trained personnel and facilities without which no Medicare arrangements could be feasible."[7]

In 1949 there were expectations that Newfoundland could catch up with Canada. Miller was more realistic and argued that catching up meant "massive increase in the infrastructure, funding, and economic development, more than Newfoundland could provide."[8] Still, the NHGP did open the door for the provincial Department of Health, enabling it to do things which otherwise would have been impossible. One incident in the operations of the programs reveals that Miller did not allow his personal opinions to override his obligation to be fair and to provide the Minister with the information he needed to arrive at a decision, even if it would be a decision he disliked. Shortly after Confederation the Minister proposed the appointment of an advisory committee to the Health Planning Committee. Miller replied that "he was not enthusiastic about the proposal," but for the Minister's guidance he enclosed material on the New Brunswick Advisory Committee.[9]

As the years passed, Miller began to experience the negative side of the programs. The provinces found irksome the continuous detailed federal control of projects and the addition of restrictions without consultation.[10] Then in August 1952, Jackson advised Miller that funding for hospitals would be cut in half.[11] Miller in his acknowledgment, has this to say about the grants in general: "It is important to lay down at the beginning that the amount for continued service will be limited and that eventually the Provincial government will have to bear part of the costs of new programs . . . I can see all kinds of trouble ahead of us when we try to transfer costs of projects initiated under federal health grants. As a matter of fact I tried it in our 1951 – 1952 estimates but with no success."[12] Here Miller put his finger on the adverse consequences of so many federal intrusions into the health care field which, by the British North America Act of 1867, is under provincial jurisdiction. Ottawa is only too happy to see itself as providing seed money for projects and then leaving the provinces to bear their ongoing operational costs. The program ended when The Royal Commission on Health Services recommended that the NHGP be replaced by a Medical Services Grant to each province as an inclusive grant to provide for disbursements to cover all aspects of medicare.[13]

One provision of the grants program merits closer attention. When it was set up the program earmarked funds for a nation- wide health survey of current health programs with a view to making recommendations for their improvement. Each province was responsible for arranging its portion of the survey. One of the last acts of the Commission of Government, in response to a request from the Canadian High Commissioner to Newfoundland, was to appoint a health planning committee with Miller as its advisor.[14] After Newfoundland joined Canada this committee was replaced by a new Committee chaired by Miller. The committee took five years to complete its task, releasing its report in 1956.[5] It contained nine recommendations. Since presumably these reflect Millers thoughts on the future of health services, the salient points are worth noting.

The first recommendation, outlining how the Department of Health should be organized, had already been implemented but tacked on to it was a plea for funding for planning and future developments as well as for the collection of statistics. The Commissioners noted that health services were too centralized with no delegation of administrative responsibility to lower levels of authority. The Commissioners expressed a hope now that local self-government was beginning to be implemented, it might be possible to pass on responsibility for a measure of health care to lower levels of authority. However, the Commissioners were realists and thought that local councils might be too busy with other tasks to be saddled with health care. Not said by the Commission, but what Miller repeated on many occasions, was the dearth of responsible, informed citizens in the remoter areas of the province from whom to select local Boards. The second recommendation was what would now be called a pilot community health centre. The third and fourth recommendations dealt with public health and advocated, amongst other measures, steps to reduce maternal and infant mortality and to control tuberculosis. The fifth recommendation stated that another 800 active treatment beds and 800 to 1000 beds for mental illness would be required by 1960 and that the older hospitals needed to be modernized and expanded. The seventh recommendation called for an extension of the bursary system to other health professional trainees besides medical and dental students*. The eighth and ninth addressed the topic of universal health care plans.The Commissioners pointed out that while almost half the population of Newfoundland was already covered, such a scheme had stretched government's reserves to their limit and was inadequate to meet the

* Some medical and dental students, "who agreed to practice in less attractive areas," had received financial assistance as far back as 1945.[15]

demands put on it. The extension of universal health care to the rest of the population should be deferred until the resources to meet the increased demand were in place. They also pointed out that collections from the subscribers to the cottage hospital system left a deficit, small it was true, but one which would be enlarged by extending universal health care to the whole population.

Looking back, we can now see that there were some striking omissions. There is no reference to rehabilitation, nor to chronic, extended, and home care. Critics might argue that the number of extra hospital beds required was inflated but, in defence of the Commissioners, tuberculosis was only beginning to come under control and out-patient psychiatric treatment was in its infancy.

Chapter 6 – Notes

1. PANL GN26/7/1.

2. PANL GN26/7/1 LAM to CHP 1949-06-01.

3. PANL GN26/7/2 FWG to LAM 1949-02-07.

4. *The Royal Commission on Health Services - Summary of Brief by NMA.* Newfoundland Medical Association Newsletter 4(11)5-71961.

5. CNS Newfoundland. Health Survey Committee. *Newfoundland Health Survey Report.* Chairperson L.A. Miller 1956.

6. PANL GN26/7/2 FWG to LAM 1950-03-14.

7. Miller L. *Medicare.* Newfoundland Journal of Commerce 35(2):28-31,38 1968.

8. Suttie Boyd Personal Communication.

9. PANL GN 26/7/1 LAM to JRC 1949- 10-05.

10. *The Royal Commission on Health Services. Submission of the Government of Newfoundland.* Newfoundland Medical Association Newsletter (3):7-9 1962 .

11. PANL GN26/7/2 FWG to LAM 1952-08-14.

12. PANL GN26/7/2 LAM to FWG 1952 08-29.

13. *Recommendations on the Royal Commission on Health Services*, News and Views. Canadian Medical Association #82 1 August 1964.

14. PANL GN26/7/1 LAM Memo 1949-01- 18.

15. Miller L. *Placement Incentives*, (Letter) Canadian Medical Association Journal 126: 120 1982.

CHAPTER 7

Children's Health Plan and Federal/Provincial Hospital Insurance

Children's Health Plan

On 22 December 1958, during a radio and television Christmas address, Premier Smallwood announced a Children's Health Plan to provide free medical and dental care for children up to their sixteenth birthday.[1] The announcement came out of the blue. There had been no prior consultation with the Department of Health or the NMA before dropping this bombshell. It was one of Smallwood's typical impulsive gestures taken on the spur of the moment without considering the costs or the adequacy of the facilities to provide the services promised by the plan. The reasons for the announcement were not clear since forty percent of the population was already receiving comprehensive care under the Cottage Hospital scheme. The beneficiaries of the plan therefore would be children in St. John's and a few larger towns. The costs would have to be borne entirely by the province. Prudence should have restrained him from taking such far-reaching steps until the government had received and examined the Health Survey Committee's report which was in preparation.* This and other unilateral ventures of Smallwood into the field of health frustrated attempts at developing long range health plans during his premiership. The Premier's announcement had taken everyone by surprise including the NMA

* It was released in the next year (see Ch. 6)

and it was left to the embarrassed Minister of Health and his Deputy Minister to deal with the resentment of the NMA and yet enlist its cooperation.

Being a minister in a Smallwood Cabinet was not an enviable post. This same Minister, Dr. J. McGrath, had no illusions about his position and used to say to Miller, "You don't for a moment think that I am really Minister of Health." What he meant of course was that Smallwood was the Minister of Health as he was Minister of most other departments.[2] He treated his Ministers like office boys. The Children's Health Plan was to be introduced in stages. The first phase, free hospitalization and in-patient diagnostic services, was introduced 1 January 1957 with the reluctant support of the NMA.[1] The expected increased demand for beds for children did not materialize,[3] probably because there was no financial incentive for physicians to admit elective cases. This was to change in December 1957 when once again without any prior discussion with the NMA, the Premier announced the implementation of the second phase of the plan, the payment of professional fees for the care of in-patients. Meanwhile, during the first phase, the NMA had requested Dr. C. Joy to conduct an assessment of hospital facilities and diagnostic services in the province. His investigations revealed inadequate numbers of beds, overcrowding and insufficiencies in diagnostic facilities.[4] The Association argued that while it was bad enough to introduce phase one with inadequate facilities, it was still more reprehensible for the government to go ahead with phase two having done nothing to increase the number of hospital beds nor to upgrade diagnostic services. Once again the Minister and his deputy had to smooth ruffled feathers and get at least a modicum of cooperation from the Association. McGrath and Miller felt called upon to remind the resentful executive officers of the Association of certain political facts of life that while they personally would never be guilty of the discourtesy of introducing new schemes without consulting the NMA, they could not vouch for their superiors.[5] However objectionable it might seem to the NMA, the Premier had acted within his rights in making the announcement . McGrath then went on to point out that he could act only as directed by the Executive Council (the Cabinet) and that if he made commitments they could be overruled. Miller chimed in that his also were subject to the same constraints.

Implementation of phase two was to cause more headaches than phase one. Negotiations for a fee schedule with the NMA were contentious.[6] Eventually agreement was reached for payment at 80 percent of the 1956 NMA schedule of fees for the first 30 days and thereafter at 40 percent. The government, foreseeing that under this schedule payments to individual pediatricians might be unacceptably high, had insisted on including a clause in the final agreement providing for a review of payment schedules after six months. By June 1958 it was obvious that this was needed. Negotiations were reopened and again agreement was difficult to reach but eventually both parties accepted the principal that after a pediatrician had received a stipulated amount from the plan he would collect only 25 percent of the agreed fee for the remainder of the contract year.[7] The plan seems to have run reasonably smoothly after that but the fee schedule had to be renegotiated from time to time.

What did Miller think of the plan, or rather the two phases that were implemented? Some years later he claimed that during the first phase there was an increase in collection rates by physicians but did not indicate the magnitude of the increase.[8] Presumably, it was because parents were able to pay professional fees now that they did not have to pay for their children's hospitalization. He put down in writing his thoughts about the plan, but in guarded terms because he was still Deputy Minister.[9] He noted that, as expected, in phase two there was a dramatic increase of admissions of children for elective operations. This was at the expense of adult admissions. Competition between children and adults for too few beds could have become a source of friction but for the introduction of the Federal/Provincial free hospitalization for all the population on 1 July 1958. The ratio of adult to pediatric hospital admissions then soon returned to what it had been before the Children's Health Plan.

Another grievance was from the the Cottage Hospital physicians who, being salaried, were debarred from collecting fees under the Plan. To satisfy their complaints the government assigned them extra pay for seeing children. The most serious defect, or "anomaly," as Miller euphemistically called it, to the Plan was " the bonus – for treatment as an in-patient rather than as an out-patient."[9] Miller used to say that when it came to phasing in universal health care in Canada, the government had started with the most expensive component, free hospitalization, rather than commencing at the cheaper other end to cover home and office visits and then expanding into more expensive areas. Obviously such a sequence would have discouraged over-utilization of hospital beds, but it overlooked the widely accepted notion that it was hospitalization which was so costly for lower middle class people, and it was this perception which was impelling politicians down the road to free hospitalization.

Miller addressed this rhetorical question: "What good has all this [The Children's Health Plan] done?"[9] He concluded that it was too early (i.e. 1960) to judge, but the plan did "show that it is possible to give one segment of medical care to one group of the population on a basis acceptable to a high proportion of all parties involved, and to do so under a department of government." Hardly a high recommendation! He also thought that the plan had probably enabled some children to receive treatment who otherwise would not have been so fortunate. Certainly the impression his paper leaves is one of unenthusiastic tolerance of the plan. His role as a Civil Servant was to see that it functioned smoothly and to gather statistics so that the plan could be evaluated periodically. This never happened because the plan was overtaken by subsequent events, first by Federal/Provincial Hospitalization Insurance (which absorbed hospitalization and diagnostic costs) and then by comprehensive medicare.

The Children's Health Plan stands out as the one innovative feature of health care during the Smallwood era. Still the question remains, "Why the rush?" since it was implemented when Federal/Provincial Hospitalization was in the offing. The impression is that the plan was dreamed up by Smallwood on the spur of the moment and from purely political considerations. It certainly put an extra strain on already inadequate facilities and insufficient personnel.

Federal/Provincial Hospital Insurance

In the years following World War II there had been discussions about a Canada-wide universal health plan and by the mid 1950s, the Dominion Government had indicated that all that delayed its implementation was the consent of the majority of the provinces. However, the provinces argued that it should be phased in with free hospitalization and diagnostic services before moving on to free ambulatory care.[10] This course was adopted because it was the cost of hospital care for people of moderate means which was creating the clamor for government funded health care. With Federal/Provincial Health Insurance slated to take effect in July 1958, the Newfoundland Minister of Health was concerned that the health infrastructure might be unable to meet the increased demand that would be placed upon it. He pushed for additional beds and an increase in the salaries of full time medical employees for fear of losing them.[11] Miller was one of those who benefited from the request. His salary was raised from ten thousand five hundred and sixty dollars to eleven thousand dollars per annum. Federal/provincial Hospital Insurance was funded on a cost-shared basis (63–37 in 1961) by the Federal and Provincial governments.

The Children's Health Plan and Federal/Provincial Hospital Insurance opened up the question of what to do about Cottage Hospital premiums. In all fairness they should have been reduced, but since they were small initially and the increase over the years had been marginal, the government elected to leave them as they were, arguing that the premium was payment for professional services covered by the Children's Health Act, but not by the Federal/Provincial Hospital Insurance scheme. In a memorandum to the Minister, Miller expressed his amazement and disappointment that Newfoundland was the only province to fund its share of the program out of general revenue rather than through a special tax or premium.[12] As a consequence Government was tardy in reimbursing the private hospitals for the cost of Federal/Provincial Hospital Insurance, forcing them to take out loans and to pay the interest themselves.

Chapter 7 – Notes

1. Knowling, T.A. *Five Point Program for Children.* Canadian Hospital 39 (2): 54-5 1962.

2. NRC Miller, L. Memoir. Unpublished.

3. ANLMA NMA Ex Comm. 1958-1-4.

4. ANLMA NMA Ex Comm. 1957-12-16.

5. ANLMA NMA Ex Comm. Undated.

6. ANLMA NMA Ex Comm. 1958-01-06.

7. ANLMA Annual Report Ex Comm. May 1959.

8. Miller, L.A. *Medicare.* Newfoundland Journal of Commerce. 35 (2): 28-31, 38 1968.

9. Miller, L.A. *The Children's Health Plan in Newfoundland.* Canadian Journal of Public Health 51(10): 385-388 1960.

10. CNS JRSC Hefferton SJ Memo 1956-02-09.

11. CNS JRSC McGrath J. Memo. Undated.

12. IRC LAM to J McG 1959-10-5.

CHAPTER 8

The Dr. Charles A. Janeway Child Health Centre

"The only serious disagreement I had with the Premier was over the proposed Children's Hospital," wrote Miller many years later.[1] For Smallwood, with his usual resort to hyperbole, the Children's Health Centre was " one of the most glorious achievements of Confederation."[2] Smallwood goes on to say "that it was a battle royal that I had to fight— the whole of the medical profession with two or three exceptions was opposed. Even the medical men in our own Department of Health were opposed. Almost to a man they wanted a wing added to the General Hospital to look after the children. One man was my immovable advisor, and inspiration, Dr. Clifford Joy. He, with great patience and skill, educated me about children's hospitals."[2] Smallwood saw himself as a knight in shining armour triumphing over tremendous odds. How did such a marked divergence develop between the Premier and the Department of Health?

By the middle of the century there were pediatric wards at the three St. John's hospitals, but by then the climate of opinion was changing. Children were best treated, so it was claimed, in hospitals dedicated entirely to their care and only this way could the specialty of pediatrics develop. Rightly or wrongly the precedent set by the Hospital for Sick Children in Great Ormond Street, London, was hard to resist and was being followed in other large centres. This view had its supporters in Newfoundland. In 1956 a committee of the NMA had recommended a Children's Hospital of 250 to 300 beds.

No steps were taken to implement this proposal. What brought things to a head was the impending transfer of the American base of Fort Pepperell in St. John's to Canadian federal and provincial authorities, slated for 10 August 1961. One of the buildings on the base was the Fort Pepperell Hospital. The Minister of Health asked the NMA to appoint a committee to advise him on its disposal. Under the chairmanship of Dr. A.E. Shapter the committee presented several options including that of a children's hospital, but ended by recommending that the building be used as a children's rehabilitation center and adult convalescent hospital.[3] This recommendation pleased the Minister, although the two pediatricians on the committee had expressed the opinion that their preference would have been a recommendation for a children's hospital. Once again the government took no action.

Shortly afterwards one of the two dissenting pediatricians, Dr. C. Joy, went into politics as a Liberal (the same party to which Smallwood belonged) and was elected to the legislature. There he began to lobby for turning Fort Pepperell Hospital into a children's hospital. He soon won Smallwood's ear and became his advisor on a children's hospital. Smallwood had already given a pledge to provide a Children's Hospital for St. John's.[4] In 1962, at Joy's suggestion, Smallwood asked Dr.Charles Janeway, a well -known Boston pediatrician, to advise him on whether Fort Pepperell Hospital could be transformed into a children's hospital. After inspecting the building, Janeway recommended that it be so used.[5] About this time the Medical Advisory Council (MAC) of the General Hospital recommended construction of a children's hospital as an adjunct to the General Hospital, citing the cost saved by sharing ancillary services.[6] The NMA had also advocated this solution.[7] As for Fort Pepperell, the MAC said that it should become a convalescent hospital, the recommendation favoured by the Department of Health.

Smallwood was placed in a dilemma. Should he follow Janeway's advice or that of the MAC of the General Hospital which was indeed the preference of his own Department of Health? The department claimed, rightly as it turned out, that it would be more costly to change Fort Pepperell into a children's hospital than to build on or adjacent to the General Hospital. Smallwood's solution to the conflicting advice he was getting was to write to Janeway and professors of pediatrics across Canada, as well as to leading pediatricians in the U.K. and the U.S.A., placing the two recommendations before them and asking which one each favoured.[4 & 8] They all recommended a pediatric hospital, distant from an adult hospital and an overwhelming majority thought, from the information given to them, that Fort Pepperell could be converted without too much expense to a Children's Hospital.

As Miller wrote, quoting a witticism of the day, "This was like asking a musician should you have a music room in your house, naturally he would say yes."[1] Smallwood got the answers he wanted and expected.

The NMA still adhering to its original recommendation protested to Miller and was told, "Don't blame me, it's not my job to make policy." In August 1966 the Fort Pepperell Hospital, now transformed at great cost into the Dr. Charles A. Janeway Child Health Centre, commonly called the "Janeway", was officially opened by Janeway before a gala audience.[5] It was the first government-owned hospital to have a Board of Governors.

Nowadays the need for austerity has forced governments to rethink their commitment to freestanding pediatric hospitals and Miller's and the NMA's warnings have been vindicated.

Chapter 8 – Notes

1. NRC Miller, L.A. Memoir. Unpublished.

2. Smallwood, J.R. *I Chose Canada* MacMillan and Company Ltd.Toronto 1977 p. 379.

3. ANLMA NMA Fort Pepperell Committee, April 1961.

4. CNS JRSC JRS to WLC 1964-1-31.

5. *Charles A. Janeway Child Health Centre Opens.* Newfoundland Medical Association Newsletter 8:6-7 1966.

6. CNS JRSC MAC General to JMcG 1964-01-29.

7. ANLMA ARM to LAM 1963-01-31.

8. CNS JRSC CJ to JRS 1964-2-4.

CHAPTER 9

The Royal Commission on Health Services

(The Hall Commission)

In June 1960, at its annual meeting, the CMA passed the statement: "The highest standard of medical services should be available to every resident of Canada. Insurance to prepay costs of medical services should be available to all regardless of age, state of health, or financial status. Certain individuals require assistance to pay medical services insurance costs." [2]

The key points of this resolution lie in the second and third clauses whereby it is clear the CMA was advocating that those who could pay for their own insurance should continue to do so and those who couldn't or who needed assistance should be subsidized in total or in part.

Shortly afterwards an official request from the association was sent to the Federal Government requesting a Royal Commission to study the health needs and resources of Canada.[3] The government responded by appointing a Royal Commission commonly referred to as the Hall Commission after its chairman, Mr. Justice E.M. Hall, to conduct a wide-ranging inquiry into the health services of the country and to recommend measures for their improvement. The Royal Commission travelled across the country holding hearings and receiving briefs. Its report was released in June 1964.

In Newfoundland it received a number of briefs from interested parties. One was from the Provincial Government. Apart from a few word changes, it was identical to the draft Miller submitted to the Minister of Health, Dr. J. McGrath.[4] Conforming to Miller's custom it was brief, but with an offer to submit additional information should it be required. Miller was a realist and understood if he had a case to make, he had to do it concisely, otherwise he ran the risk of losing his reader's attention. In a short preamble he painted a dismal picture of the Newfoundland health scene, noting that by such indices of health as infant mortality and tuberculosis death rates, Newfoundland was far behind other parts of Canada. Outpatient facilities and hospital beds for taking care of the physically and mentally ill were either unsatisfactory or insufficient or both. Professional personnel were too few in spite of a bursary program to support medical and dental students.

Arising out of this background information there were five recommendations. Having discussed where to begin when all facets of Health Care, other than private practice, were in such a deplorable state, Miller recommended the infusion of extra funds at every level. Consequently, the first recommendation was that Newfoundland be given "special consideration" by the federal authorities and be provided with funds to upgrade all government-operated health services. The second, reflecting frustration and irritation with the rigid control down to the most minute detail exercised by Ottawa over the NHGP, suggested an inquiry aimed at introducing a much looser and less cumbersome oversight. The third related to the student bursary program which was a significant charge on the treasury. The brief noted that the training requirements for health professionals were steadily increasing in length which thus was adding to the costs of the programs. Consequently, the government recommended that the Royal Commission conduct an inquiry to see if training programs could be shortened without affecting quality. He was farsighted in making this novel suggestion. In essence what he was advocating was an inquiry to see if the amount of time required to meet the objectives of educational programs for health professionals could be shortened by what would now be designated as evidence-based studies – a plea that was to go as unheeded then as now. The fourth recommendation was a plea to increase federal hospital construction grants to more realistic levels and to expand the federal/provincial hospitalization program to include mental and tuberculosis patients. The fifth and final recommendation, foreseeing some form of medicare, recommended that the Department of Health be charged with its administration. Miller was vigilant in guarding the prerogatives of his department and quick to react when he sensed that there might be attempts to strip it of what he considered to be its legitimate tasks.

In contrast to the government brief, the NMA presentation[5] was longer but, with a few exceptions, there does not appear to be any fundamental difference between the department and the NMA in their philosophies of health care. Both showed the same concern at the inadequacies of health services and the need for more beds for the physically and mentally ill; but in addition, the NMA brief drew attention to the need to provide facilities for convalescent care and rehabilitation, a surprising omission in the government brief unless its first recommendation, by implication, included these areas. The department's brief made no reference to nursing services, while the NMA brief advocated two more hospital-based nursing schools. The two briefs also differed on their observations on the Cottage Hospital system. The government in its original submission confined itself to listing its deficiencies. On the other hand the NMA brief referred to the high turnover rate of medical staff compared to private practitioners in the larger centres. The NMA's antidote was to extend private practice into the Cottage Hospital regions, funded by a mixture of personal health insurance and government subsidies. This would require the institution of local boards to determine the rates of capitation fees and government subsidies to practitioners.

A major difference of opinion between the NMA and the department surfaced over this recommendation. The department argued that private practice had never thriven in the outposts, and that the Cottage Hospital system could be improved, with consequent less turnover, by the provision of "better facilities, higher salaries, plus pensionability and increased personnel."[6] Why the government brief had not mentioned these points in the first place is not known. Miller should have realized that the background to the department's first recommendation was far too brief, and that the Cottage Hospital system was too important yet had too many deficiencies to be buried in an all encompassing recommendation. This is an example when Miller's brevity did not stand him in good stead.

The NMA's brief had one recommendation that doesn't have so much as an echo in the department's brief or its supplementary submissions. The NMA suggested that consideration be given to establishing a medical school in St. John's, citing its beneficial effect on continuing education and opening up careers for young Newfoundlanders.[5]

What heed did the Commissioners pay to these two briefs? The first and fifth recommendations of the departments submission, were ignored, presumably because the first was pressing for special status for Newfoundland and the fifth was an internal matter for each province to settle as it saw fit. The other three resolutions crop up in the recommendations of the Commission, although the third in a somewhat watered down form (Recommendation 182).[7] In the case of the NMA brief, the proposal of a subsidized prepayment private practice in rural areas is not mentioned and could not be because of the Commission's support of universal, government-funded medicare. But the Commission did recommend that consideration be given to establishing a medical school in St. John's "if a study supported the idea."[7] The most celebrated recommendations of the Commission are those covering "Comprehensive, Universal, Personal Health Services to be funded on a 50 – 50 cost share basis between the Federal and Provincial authorities."[7]

In the weeks that followed it became clear that there was a cleavage between the CMA and the Royal Commission.[8] Perhaps by this time the CMA was wondering how wise it had been in calling for a Royal Commission in the first place. The fundamental differences are summed up in the first, second and fifth clauses of the CMA statement on the Royal Commission's Report:

> 1. The Commission has concluded that Personal Medical Services should become a social responsibility provided by the State. The CMA has always believed that Personal Health Services should be an individual responsibility for self supporting citizens.
>
> 2. The Commission recommends that public monies should be used to provide Health Services for all Canadians on a com-

pulsory basis. We believe that the monies should only be used to assist lower income groups to purchase insurance

5. The CMA believes that individuals should have a choice of coverage available from multiple carriers. Under the Commission's proposals all insuring agencies and the prepayment plans which the profession has sponsored would cease to exist."[8]

In essence the CMA was proposing that there be a minimum amount of insurance which all needed and the state should contribute only to assist those who could not pay for this minimum coverage. To support its arguments the CMA observed that 75% of Canadians were covered by their own prepaid insurance policies and of the remaining 25% only 3% encountered difficulties in paying medical bills.[9] "The idea of regimenting 100% of the public and 100% of the medical profession to cope with the happily small minority who ran into heavy expenses in any single year is neither desirable, nor logical, nor economical."[9]

The reply to these arguments was the practical difficulties of identifying those who were unable to pay for insurance in whole or in part, and of determining what should be the minimal amount of insurance coverage for these two classes. The CMA proposals, it was claimed, would have had the effect of creating a two-tiered system, a rich man's medicine and a poor man's medicine, something that was not acceptable in the egalitarian age which Canada had entered.

But in spite of these perfectly valid claims there were still Cassandra-like voices. Any scheme involving payment of doctors by government would be bound to lead to confrontation; the effect of medicare on the economy could be deleterious (government expenditures on health had risen from 21% of its budget in 1951 to 35% in 1966);[10] if this trend continued there would be reduced incentive for investing and reduced ability to compete;[11] finally, just as Medicade in the USA had had inflationary consequences, so also, they warned, would medicare.[12]

A comment from the CMA special committee examining the Hall Commission's report should be allowed to close this particular debate on medicare: "Limitless Medical Care is an unattainable ideal

. . . the simple essential problem is that a blank cheque is given to the patient for utilization and the physician for service."[13] Prophetic words that Miller used to quote with resigned forebodings to his intimates in his remaining few years as Deputy Minister.

Looking back at the medicare debate it is hard to avoid the conclusion that each side was irresistible in the offence but powerless in the defence.

Chapter 9 – Notes

1. Royal Commission on Health Services. Ottawa. Queen's Printer, 1964. Cat. no. Zl-1961/3-1

2. ANLMA Statement on Medical Services, General Council Ninety-fourth Annual Meeting. Canadian Medical Association June 1960.

3. ANLMA News and Views. Canadian Medical Association July 11, 1964. No. 80.

4. CNS Miller, Leonard. *A Brief for Submission to the Royal Commission on Health Services* submitted to the Honourable James McGrath Minister of Health 1961.

5. ANLMA Submission to the Royal Commission on Health Services by the Newfoundland Medical Association. 1961-11-02

6. ANLMA Comments [by the Newfoundland Department of Health] on Submission of Newfoundland Division Canadian Medical Association. (Including Exhibit 23 A).

7. ANLMA News and Views, Canadian Medical Association August 1, 1964 No. 82.

8. *CMA Policy on the Hall Commission.* Newfoundland Medical Association Newsletter 6 (5):7 1964 .

9. ANLMA Catherwood, R. *Real Medicare Fights Still Over Costs and Rights – Not the Date.* Financial Post September 17, 1966.

10. ANLMA Hockin TA *Canada: Welfare or Insurance State* Published in Executive August 1966.

11. ANMLA The Interpretor N8 March 1967 Published by Canadian Health Insurance Association 1303 Yonge St. Toronto, Canada.

12. ANMLA *The Economics of Health* (*The Morgan Guaranty Survey* May 1967) A CMA Economics Newsletter 1966-10-6.

13. *Statement on Medical Care With Conclusions and Recommendations, Special Committee on Policy of the Canadian Medical Association.* Canadian Medical Association Journal 91(12) Special Supplement pg. 14. 1964.

CHAPTER 10

Medicare

The Federal Government, despite warnings from the CMA,[1] chose to follow the path recommended by the Royal Commission on Health Services and proceeded to pass the Medical Care Act of Canada in 1966 to take affect on 1 July 1968. Under the terms of the Act the Government offered to pay 50% of per capita costs to any province which enacted a medical care insurance scheme which had the four attributes of universality, comprehensiveness, portability and which was administered by a non-profit agency.

The federal offer was far too attractive for the provinces to ignore. Although it was only a matter of time before each signed up, the merits and drawbacks of Ottawa's proposal continued to be the subject of a heated debate. All were agreed that every Canadian was entitled to comprehensive health care regardless of financial circumstances, but arguements continued over the methods of funding and extent of care. Was it to be a system, as recommended by the CMA, funded through payment by citizens of insurance premiums, the extent of coverage depending on the size of the premiums, with the government assisting those unable to pay the premiums for a minimum amount of coverage? Or was it, as proposed by the Hall Commission, to be a comprehensive, universal system funded by government regardless of individuals' financial circumstances?

Miller expressed his views in an article on medicare before it was implemented.[2] His purpose was to enlighten the public and it is written in his usual dispassionate style. The content is factual and it brings out the arguments of both sides of the debate without taking sides. He takes the story of medicare back to World War II and the Federal Advisory Committee on Health Insurance, the time when governments of the Western world, particularly the United Kingdom, were devoting themselves to planning for a better world after victory. Universal, comprehensive health care was one of these goals. Miller liked to bring issues back to first principals .

The most important of these was financial. Echoing the stand of the CMA he asked, "Why should governments provide everybody benefits which large amounts of the population can and now do successfully provide for themselves?" Then, siding with the proponents of the Hall Commission, he asks if there was to be a means test to determine who could and who could not pay. He then takes up the question of a one- versus a two-tiered system and wonders whether medicare should cover all medical services or provide for only a basic degree of care. He reminds his readers there had never been a tradition of local self-government in Newfoundland and consequently the Government of the day had been forced to shoulder the cost of health services for the outports since the turn of the century – a kind of "Miniature Medicare" in his words. Now medicare was coming along and providing the monies for the province to operate health services which had become a strain on the provincial purse. However, it would be foolish, he said, to forget that while the present financial aspects of the plan were attractive, inevitably the province might be obliged to shoulder an increasingly higher proportion of the costs.

Here he was in agreement with Smallwood. The Premier, according to one of his ministers of health,[3] had the same reservations about medicare and had asked the federal authorities what guarantee was there that they would continue to adhere to the proposal of funding on a 50-50 basis. His forebodings were not put to rest by bland assurances that he need have no fears on this score. Miller concluded with these words: "Medicare, another and eventually costly link in the chain of social services has many of the same advantages and disadvantages of the links already in operation, it should spread the cost of illness and relieve many people of the crippling costs now possible. It will be abused as other programs – which will decrease to the extent that a sense of responsibility can be engendered in the individual to any government financed operations."[2]

As far back as 1965, anticipating medicare, the Department of Health entered into informal discussions with the NMA on matters that needed to be settled prior to their implementation, such as overdemand for insufficient services, unnecessary utilization, payments to salaried physicians and mechanisms for coping with unacceptably high disbursements.[4,5,6]

In the autumn of 1967, Miller sent a lengthy memorandum to the new Minister of Health, John Crosbie, enumerating the items for which decisions were required before medicare legislation took effect.[7] It shows an understanding of the operations of medicare, the steps required to put it in place and a knowledge of the machinery to do so which had already been set in motion. The memorandum included two points: a suggestion that the Maritime Hospital Service Association be approached to sound out its willingness to serve as the paying agent for medicare; and a discussion of the question of retaining, as had other provinces, a firm of outside consultants to advise on the administration and organization of medicare. Miller was not enthusiastic about this last proposal. "Our policy has been not to recommend the employment of consultants based on a feeling that the cost would not be justified . . . the personnel of this department has had more experience with various types of medical care planning than those in other provinces except Saskatchewan."

The Minister seems to have used this memorandum as the basis for one of his own to the cabinet to obtain approval on the most urgent items.[8] The first was the funding of medicare in which the minister recommended financing from general revenues. The second was the administration of medicare. The Minister argued that since his department was not equipped to take on this task, a separate agency would have to be created or possibly the Maritime Hospital Service Association might be willing to serve as the fiscal agent. The cabinet approved of the first recommendation but in the case of the second, opted for a separate commission to administer medicare, responsible to the Minister of Health. Miller was overruled on the matter of employing outside consultants and Kates Peat Marwick (KPM) was retained in October 1967.[9] Their proposed administrative organizational chart for medicare was a disappointment to both Miller and the Minister. Miller's comments are trenchant. "I'm appalled by the payments that I believe would be the results of the consultants suggestions."[10] He then goes on to add that the cost of the proposed administration could go as high as a million dollars per annum and even then not meet the major aims of medicare which must be "prompt payment of physicians and availability of early information to check unfavorable trends [i.e. excessive payments to physicians]". KPM's administrative chart, he thought, was well summed up in the Minister's own words: "The trappings of an elephant on the back of a mouse." But in spite of these harsh words, the department seems to have organized medicare along the lines proposed by KPM.[9]

Late in the year the government had second thoughts about implementing medicare by 1 July 1968. Miller warned that uncertainty was hampering planning and that if the date was to be postponed he needed to know soon.[11] Meanwhile negotiations continued with the NMA. Two contentious issues surfaced, the first relating to the fee schedule. Was remuneration to be at 100% of the current NMA fee schedule, as demanded by the NMA, or at a lower rate? The government argued that since the doctors would have no unpaid bills, remuneration should be at a lower rate than the NMA fee schedule.[9] The second item of dispute was "opting out." The NMA argued that a physician should have the right to opt out with the right to charge a higher fee than the medicare plan stipulated, provided that prior notification had been given to his patients. The patients should then have the right to claim back from the Commission the amount that medicare normally paid for the service received.[12, 13] To discourage patients from not paying opted out physicians' fees and pocketing cheques received from the government, the NMA pressed the department to have the cheques made out to both patient and physician, requiring the signatures of each for cashing.[14]

During a debate on the topic at the 1967 Annual General Meeting (AGM) of the Association, Miller insisted on going on record as being opposed to opting out because it could end in an excessively high rate of overbilling, something no government would tolerate.[15] But, as the President pointed out, this was being unrealistic. Only about one percent of the population could afford extra charges.

In 1968 an Act respecting Insured Medical Care Services to take effect on 1 April 1969 was passed by the Legislative Assembly which provided for remuneration at a yet to be decided percentage of the NMA fee schedule.[9] Opting out was also to be permitted but the government refused the NMAs request for physician and patient co-signatures of the cheque of reimbursement for the medicare share of the opted out physicians account and insisted on making out the cheque to the patient only.[14] Thus there was a financial disincentive to opting out and in fact initially only four physicians chose to do so and then opted in one by one. The reasons the Act cited for joining medicare were that it would not substantially increase government expenditures on health, provided demand did not increase too dramatically, and it would eliminate the regional inequities in payments for treating indigents. The Act also stated that the government was obliged to fund Newfoundland's portion of costs out of general revenues because if it had adopted a means test the funds it would have received from Ottawa under the Canada Assistance Plan would be less than under medicare.

After the introduction of medicare Miller's career had only two years to run but, as expected before his retirement, it became apparent that some physicians' earnings were unacceptably high. The agreement worked out between the NMA and the government (similar to the one followed in the Children's Health Plan of a ceiling on individual earnings followed by a sliding scale thereafter) was hailed as a model of government-physician cooperation in the handling of an issue that could have blown up into confrontation.[16]

Chapter 10 – Notes

1. ANLMA *Statement by The Canadian Medical Association*, Press release CMA House July 21, 1965.

2. Miller, L.A. *Medicare.* Newfoundland Journal of Comrnerce. 35(2): 28-31, 38 1968.

3. Hickman, TAH Personal Communication.

4. ANLMA J McG to WDP 1965-10-7.

5. ANLMA NMA Medicare Comm. 1966-04-07.

6. ANLMA NMA Cott. Hosp. Comrn. 1967-08-26 .

7. CNS JCCC LAM to JCC 1967-10-5.

8. CNS JCCC Health 7 (B) -' 67 JCC Memo Medicare.

9. Crosbie JC *An address made by the Minister of Health John C. Crosbie on moving second reading of the Newfoundland Medical Care Insurance Act 1968* . Newfoundland Medical Association Newsletter 10 (3):6-16 1968.

10. CNS JCCC LAM to JCC 1968-02-05.

11. CNS JCCC LAM TO JCC 1967-12-15.

12. ANLMA WDP To JCC 1968-04-17.

13. Mercer AR *The Implications of Medicare* Newfoundland Medical Association Newsletter 9 (4):8- 10 1967.

14. WDP Personal Communication.

15. Newfoundland Medical Association Newsletter 9 (3) :8 1967.

16. *Newfie Government, Doctors Set Important Example.* Toronto Globe & Mail (Editorial) 1971-3-27.

CHAPTER 11

The Royal Commission on Health[1] (The Brain Commission)

By the late 1950s dissatisfaction with the medical services in the province was widespread and becoming more vocal. Cottage Hospitals needed repairs, the staff was insufficient and overworked and the accommodations poor. In St. John's the situation at the General Hospital was equally unsatisfactory; repairs and more beds were urgently needed. The young specialists who were coming back to St. John's were becoming restive and drifting to the two private hospitals where they were finding a warmer welcome and more tangible support. McGrath and Miller were widely blamed for the deficiencies of the health care system and accused of doing nothing and being wedded to the status quo.

Behind the scene Miller was equally perturbed and put down on paper his concerns in a letter addressed to the Minister of Health, Dr. James McGrath.[2] This was a most unusual step for Miller to take. McGrath and he were long-standing friends, in and out of each other's offices every day. Only a near crisis could have induced Miller to adopt this formal method of communication. For, as he writes, "the undersigned does not believe in the policy of writing memoranda merely for the record or to shift responsibility to other shoulders, rather this is written to emphasize deficiencies in personnel and facilities in the hope that something can be done, even within the present provincial financial limitations to stop a trend which appears to be rapidly developing towards complete disintegration of many services of the Health Department." Miller listed the deficiencies in the system: the administrative staff of the department was small and had time to focus only on urgent problems; there were too few hospital beds and insufficient professional staff to service them; the morale of the cottage hospitals was low and finding and retaining professional staff was running into increasing difficulties; the Children's Hospital and Federal/Provincial Hospital programs had increased the call for services which were inadequate even before their introduction, yet little had been done to expand them to meet the increased demand; public health was equally defective, judging from experience with the recent polio immunization program.

Others also were alarmed at what was perceived as a looming deterioration in services. Dr. Ian Rusted, an internist who also was a part-time consultant with the department, felt impelled to put pen to paper in a letter to McGrath to document the system's defects, but, unlike Miller, he offered solutions.[3] He also saw the recruitment of adequate medical manpower as a major challenge. To meet it he had two remedies; an extension of the government bursary program to assist second and third year premedical and predental students, and the establishment of a medical school. For the past few years he had made it his business to collect information on medical schools and in his letter he summarized the results of his study. The time was now ripe, he argued, for the Government, the University and the NMA to cooperate and explore this option. With respect to the General Hospital, its inadequacies were spurring physicians to move to the private hospitals. He concluded by saying that with these deficiencies the department needed advice and recommended a committee of inquiry into the health services of the province.

Perhaps rumblings of discontent reached Smallwood's ears and convinced him something had to be done. His minister of health was opposed to a Royal Commission but was willing to go along with a committee of inquiry.[4] Smallwood, who made frequent visits to the UK discussed his predicament with various prominent personages there and then, without consultation with his colleagues, approached Lord Brain, a well known English neurologist who had been awarded a peerage for his services to medicine, to be a one-man Royal Commission to conduct an inquiry into all aspects of medical services in the province and to make recommendations.*

* In Smallwood's memoirs there is only one brief reference to Lord Brain relating that he was appointed to advise on a medical school.[5]

The choice of a stranger to the province to carry out such a far-reaching inquiry appears odd. His ignorance of the local scene would be a handicap and besides he was liable to become a catspaw for those pushing their own pet schemes. But there is a simpler explanation for Smallwood's choice, for he was an ardent Anglophile with a special fascination for a peer of the realm. It was gratifying to flamboyantly announce that an English peer with a world-wide reputation had accepted his invitation to come and pinpoint the deficiencies of Newfoundland's health care system and to come up with remedies.

Unfortunately, it wasn't as simple as that. It was pointed out to Smallwood that he had either forgotten or had chosen to ignore the fact that feasibility studies for a medical school were well under way and that Lord Brain's mandate overlapped these activities.[4] Smallwood was a bit taken aback when he was reminded of this duplication with all its dangers of a clash. He sensibly left it up to Rusted and the university to work out a *modus operandi* with Lord Brain and it is a credit to the good sense of all concerned that they were able to do so; Lord Brain wisely staying out of the university's feasibility studies but availing himself of the results of their labours.

Russell Brain toured the province and received briefs from interested parties, including one from the Department of Health, presumably drafted by Miller.[6] In its brief the department dwelt on the well recognized inadequacies of the health services, the competition between the Department of Health and other departments for scarce dollars, and emphasis on curative medicine to the neglect of preventive health. Concern was expressed that medicare, when it came, would put a further strain on services already stretched to the limit. It would also widen the gap in income between the salaried physicians and those in private practice, making it more difficult to recruit for rural regions. No one could disagree with these observa tions but of great significance, and for the first time, the department came out publicly in favour of a medical school.

Another proposal was for a reallocation of the health budget to favour preventive rather than curative programs. A master plan for construction of new hospitals and renovation of the old was urgently required to replace the haphazard system of assigning responsibilities for building and maintenance to Public Works while saddling the Department of Health with the task of finding the funds to operate them. The General Hospital required enlargement and renovation if it was to become a teaching hospital for a Newfoundland medical school. The time had now come to assign beds for convalescent and rehabilitation purposes. Facilities were needed for retarded children. A number of recommendations concerned government - salaried physicians. To attract and retain practitioners in rural regions their salaries should be raised and the doctors should be incorporated into the Civil Service which would make them eligible for pensions. Opportunities for postgraduate education should be available and accommodations improved. Financial provision was also required to attract recruits into ancillary health professions. Looking back there does not appear to be any serious omission from the department's shopping list, except that occupational and environmental medicine and home care are neglected entirely.

Lord Brain's report was published in three volumes in 1966.[1] He must have been impressed by the Department of Health's brief, because all its recommendations crop up in one form or another in his list of proposals. His recommendations stem from the deficiencies that he perceived in the system. There was a shortage of medical manpower and Newfoundland was behind the mainland in medical technology and in specialist representation. He favoured establishing a medical school because it would go a long way towards remedying these two deficiencies. Another fault of the system was organizational stagnation. Administratively speaking, things were the same as in 1934. He did not spell out precisely what he meant by this indictment, but he seems to be referring to the over-centralization and paternalism that had been the reigning philosophy since the Royal Commission of 1930. As a consequence, there was no public involvement in policy making or in the administration of health services and facilities.

To remedy these defects, influenced perhaps by the NMA brief, Lord Brain proposed decentralization and public participation. A provincial health council with broad representation from the health professions and the public should be constituted as an advisory and consultative body to the Minister of Health. To bring in the public, he recommended regional health boards consisting of local and government-nominated representatives to whom the task of the day-to-day running of the health services within their regions would be delegated. Smallwood, it is said, had hoped that the report would favour regionalization of health services.[7] The government-owned hospitals should have similarly constituted boards.

Lord Brain recognized the inefficiencies arising form the division of responsibility for the provision of health services between three government departments (health, public works, and supply) and in his ninth recommendation proposed that "the department of health should be responsible for all aspects of the health services including the building of new hospitals and the extension and maintenance of existing ones. All present responsibilities resting with public works and other departments in these matters, should be transferred to the department of health which should have a multi discipline team to work as a planning and development section of the department." The implications of this recommendation was to prove a major problem of interpretation.

Brain did not spare the Department of Health from criticism. It was so busy attending to day-to-day matters that it had no time for long-term planning. For example, although there was a health planning committee it had met for the first time as late as August 1965.

Lord Brain came to the extraordinary conclusion that the title Deputy Minister was misleading and implied that the incumbent was an elected politician. Consequently, he proposed replacing the Deputy Minister by two officials, a Chief Medical Officer, charged with the task of advising the Minister on health matters and, co-equal with him, a lay person as Chief Secretary responsible for their implementation. It is claimed that Lord Brain thought that physician administrators could not be trusted to disburse public funds wisely and therefore their power to do so should be limited.

What did Miller think of Lord Brains labours? Not too highly, even though the latter had extensively endorsed the Department's brief, judging from a memorandum Miller sent the Minister of Health expressing his opinions.[8] "In many ways the report is disappointing, the Department of Health is given but scant recognition for what it has achieved." He points out the dilemma facing civil servants, when government appoints a commission of inquiry into the performance of their department. "The department was at a disadvantage in that the full story could not be told. Because of uncertainty concerning the method of presentation of the brief from the department and because it was not deemed advisable publicly to criticize government policies, the department was unable to present an effective case."

Miller then comments on the recommendations of the report. Naturally he concurred with those recommendations which had been proposed in the province's brief and to which he had been a major contributor. He dismissed the proposal to divide the Deputy Minister's duties between a Chief Medical Officer and a Chief Secretary as "unworkable." Regarding the proposal for regional health boards, Miller observed that their success would depend on "a willingness of government 1) to delegate authority, and 2) the availability of suitable people." He ended pessimistically that "experience of town councils is not encouraging." On the other hand he saw no problem in the appointment of Boards for the General Hospital and the Hospital for Mental and Nervous Diseases because both were located in St. John's where there were businessmen eminently qualified to serve and where there was a long tradition of self-government.

Looking at the report as a whole, Miller could not help but being struck by the realization that many of the recommendations would require a complete reorganization of the department for their implementation. Furthermore, the Deputy Minister, instead of being the final channel of communication between the Minister and the Department, would be bypassed in many instances. He saw three other defects in the report: lack of emphasis on public health and preventive medicine, omission of the problem of tuberculosis and too much faith in the value of boards. The first and second charges hardly seem justified, and tuberculosis had ceased to be a major problem. But Miller's lack of enthusiasm for boards rested on more solid ground and requires more extensive discussion.

Miller was a creature of his times. He had received his training in public health and administration in the Puddester-Mosdell era with its firmly held belief that in times of hardship with limited financial resources at hand, only a strong central authority could deliver health services efficiently and at low cost. It is true the Health and Public Welfare Act of 1931 created a medical council for the General hospital but this was purely an advisory committee.[9] The act also gave the department the authority to appoint at its own discretion local boards of heath with the district MHO as chairman. But these had only the limited function of promulgating public health regulations for their districts.

The philosophy of central control of health services persisted well into the Smallwood era. Since the system gave the government ample opportunity to exercise patronage, this is probably the explanation of Smallwood's resistance to the appointment of an administrative board for the General Hospital. It may then seem somewhat inconsistent that he was agreeable to the appointment of an administrative board for the Janeway Children's Hospital and favoured the regionalization recommended in Lord Brain's report, but perhaps by this time (the mid-1960s) he realized it would be politically unwise to resist the rising tide, demanding public participation in the administration of government-operated health services.

Practically the whole of Miller's career as a civil servant was played out against this backdrop of rigid central control of health services and only in his last years did the first steps towards loosening the reins begin. Essentially his acceptance of boards was pragmatic and like Smallwood's evolved with the passage of time, but for more credible reasons. Surprisingly, he himself was a member of only two statutory boards, one advisory and the other administrative at a privately owned hospital. The first was the Medical Council, later renamed the Medical Advisory Council (MAC) of the General hospital of which he was *ex officio* chairman. His performance there will be discussed later (Ch. 14). The second board on which he sat, was the board of the Western Memorial Hospital, a private hospital in Corner Brook. Presumably his membership of this board was by invitation and a consequence of a hospital by-law. On at least one occasion his membership of that board was to cause him embarrassment. No doubt his training and experiences on both these boards coloured his opinions. He seems to have been especially skeptical of the usefullness of advisory committees.[10] It was not that he resented advice; far from it. But he preferred to seek it within the privacy of an office on a one-to-one basis.

His reservations about administrative boards at government-funded institutions were stronger. He seems to have taken no trouble to conceal them and probably they formed the basis of the accusations of hostility towards them. One recently returned young specialist on the staff of the General hospital who was lobbying for a board in the 1950s, recalls him saying: "Over my dead body." His opinions were essentially utilitarian and he used to say to his assistants: "If government has to provide funds for an institution, why add an extra layer bureaucracy." He also realized that boards entailed a diminution of government control. He realized though, that they had their uses. They relieved the government of the responsibility of the day-to-day running of institutions and had a propaganda value by giving the impression of public involvement in their administration. He was perfectly willing to accept a hospital board when a good case could be made for its value.[11]

After the introduction of federal/provincial hospital insurance in 1958, boards at the private hospitals began to lose their autonomy as their activities became circumscribed by the funds and the terms of the grants they received from government. Unionization of their staff accelerated the process. By the end of Miller's career, their role and authority were no different than those of boards at the two government-owned hospitals – the Janeway and the General hospital –which had been constituted in 1966 and 1969 respectively.

The curtailment of freedom of action of boards at the privately owned hospitals during the last few years of Miller's career did not make for more amicable relations between them and the Department of Health. On the contrary, disputes became more frequent and more acrimonious. It is worth citing two incidents to illustrate this point. Both occurred at the private hospital where Miller was a member of the board and he was involved in both. No doubt the lessons weren't lost on hlm.

The Administrator of the Western Memorial Hospital writing to the Minister of Health, noted that a commission of inquiry into a labour dispute at the hospital had recommended a salary increase and that he had asked the Minister's consent to act upon this recommendation. The Minister wrote to Smallwood that he had replied by pointing out that personnel would be tempted to leave the Sanatorium where salaries were lower and move to the Western Memorial Hospital, and that he had enunciated the dictum that government policy had to be that "civil servant salaries are the same in any part of the province for posts of similar grade and seniority."[12] Once this guideline became established government policy, individual hospital boards could no longer participate in collective bargaining.[13]

One can sympathize with the bind in which hospital boards could find themselves, obliged to cut back services because of lack of funds, staff and the public vociferously complaining, and the government sternly warning them to live within their budgets. It is no wonder that at times they were tempted to kick over the traces, as happened once in Corner Brook.

The operating costs projected by the hospital board exceeded the budget allotted to the Western Memorial Hospital.[14] The board was reminded that the government expected the hospital to function within its allotted budget even if this meant a reduction of services and of staff. The Administrator replied in words expressing the board's frustration at being expected to provide services but without sufficient funds to do so: "As a board we are charged with the responsibility of not only providing adequate medical care to patients without our ability to provide adequate services to the people in the region depending on our hospital. Until such time as we are prevented from doing so, we intend operating the hospital in accordance with these principles even it means contravening government policy.[14,15] In his reply the Minister pointed out that the board could only operate within the grant it received from the government, and warned, "My colleagues and I are disturbed by the suggestion that your Board is prepared to disregard government policy and budgetary requirements. . . I am sure you would agree that such action . . .ultimately would reduce the hospital to insolvency. . . [and] would constitute a complete abdication of responsibility by the Board. Your Board's function and responsibility is to provide the best possible service to the public with the money available to you . . . which is what the government must do on a much wider scale."[16] Eventually, with the assistance of the Department of Health, the board was able to work out a more realistic budget and co-operative relations were restored.[17]

Miller's caution about public participation in the health care system extended beyond boards, even to well-intentioned public endeavors to raise funds to upgrade a service. A committee was formed in an outport to solicit funds for purchase of a piece of equipment. An official in the Department of Health gave his consent subject to inspection and approval by the Department of Public Works of the project on which the money was to be spent.[18] Miller was provided with an account of these activities and his approval was sought. He minuted on the margin of the memorandum that he was "not optimistic about such offers and that the Department should limit such local involvement in the Cottage Hospitals". He did not offer any reasons for his reservations. Perhaps he thought that only the Department should have the prerogative of choosing on what projects to spend money. In this case there seemed to have been ample safeguards against the squandering of money and his opinion seems unnecessarily discouraging, an attitude that could only throw cold water on voluntary public collections of money for specific purposes. For a civil servant ever conscious of straitened means one would have thought he would have welcomed contributions from the public.

One cannot help comparing the Brain Commission to the Royal Commission of Health and Public Charities (1930). The latter was to have a far-reaching impact on health services for many decades. The former was of ephemeral interest only and few of its recommendations were implemented. It is true the recommendations for boards were adopted with some enthusiasm, but this was probably to come about anyway. Feasibility studies for a medical school were well under way when Lord Brain was just an additional voice in its favour. Other recommendations were of no use because their implications for the administrative structure of the department had not been thought through. An example of Lord Brain's lack of knowledge of administrative procedures of the Government of Newfoundland appears in his ninth recommendation that the Department of Health should be given responsibility for the construction and maintenance of all hospitals. Was Lord Brain recommending that the Department of Health should go into the building trade? Miller was always careful to maintain that the problem was the lack of a long-term master plan for hospital construction and expansion and not the division of responsibilities between the Departments of Health and Public Works. For example, relations were cordial between the two departments when J.R. Chalker was moved from Health to become Minister of Public Works, a post he was to hold for twelve years. He was frequently chaffed by his deputy minister for consulting Miller on hospital construction and renovations. The person to blame for the chaos in hospital construction and maintenance was surely Smallwood. Obviously the remedy lay in a joint health and public works hospital construction and maintenance planning committee.

Interpreting the all-encompassing ninth recommendation in the Brain Commission report would have caused many headaches when it came to implementation, which fortunately did not happen. Did it mean, for example, that the purchase of medical supplies should be transferred from the Government Purchasing Agency and placed under Health?[19] Miller and his officials debated whether this was Lord Brain's intention and decided he would not have recommended such an unworkable scheme.

Lord Brain's report is open to criticism on a number of points, but in fairness he was a stranger to the province and was not a well man when he accepted Smallwood's invitation. He died shortly after the release of his report.

Chapter 11 – Notes

1. Royal Commission on Health, Right Honourable Lord Brain. Vol. 1 January 1966, Vol. 2 July 1966, Vol. 3, October 1966.Published by the Government of Newfoundland and Labrador.

2. IRC LAM to J McG 1959-10-05.

3. IRC IR to J McG 1964-09-06.

4. Rusted, I. Personal Communication.

5. Smallwood, JR, ibid. p. 385-386.

6. PANL PRC 19 Health Box 35-1-6-1, Brief by Department of Health to the Royal Commission on Health 1965-08-19.

7. Blanchard, TA. Personal Communication.

8. CNS JCCC LAM to J McG. 1966-03-24.

9. PANL Health and Public Welfare Act 1931, Acts of the General Assembly of Newfoundland.

10. PANL GN26/7/1 LAM to JRC 1949-10-5.

11. Rowe AT. *Carbonear – Blue-Print For the Future*. Newfoundland Medical Association Newsletter 6(2):12-14 1964.

12. CNS JRSC J. McG to JRS. 1964-01-13.

13. CNS EMRC Health 5-'70 ER Memo to Ex Council Health 1970-1-28.

14. CNS EMRC RJB to CAS 1969-12-15.

15. CNS EMRC LM to ER 1969-12-23.

16. CNS EMRC ER to LM 1970-1-7.

17. CNS EMRC RJB to ER 1970-1-27.

18. CNS EMRC GG to LAM 1970-1-28.

19 CNS GEC Memo. 1967-11-08.

CHAPTER 12

The Medical School

Prior to 1969, Newfoundlanders wishing to train as physicians used to enrol at one of the Medical Schools in the British Isles or on the Mainland.

By the time Miller was a student, Dalhousie University Medical School was becoming the centre attracting the greatest number of Newfoundland medical students. At the prodding of Dalhousie University, the Commission of Government agreed to start giving an annual grant towards the operating expenses of the medical school.[1] The first subvention in 1942 was set at five thousand dollars per annum, but over the years it was increased.

After Newfoundland joined Canada and the population grew and prospered, so did its ambitions to have its own educational institutions to train the professional personnel it needed.

When was serious thought given to Newfoundland's establishing its own medical school? In the late 1950s a number of St. John's physicians seriously debated the topic.[2] By 1960 discussions had advanced far enough for the NMA, in its brief to the Royal Commission on Health Services, to request the Commission to consider the idea of a medical school for Newfoundland.[3] One of the reasons cited was that there were more qualified Newfoundland premedical students than could be accommodated in medical schools across the country.

One of the physicians who had participated in the discussions, was Dr. Ian Rusted, an internist who held a part-time appointment with the government but who, in addition, was responsible for post-graduate training at the General Hospital and was Chairman of the NMA Continuing Medical Education Committee. The event which stirred him to move beyond the talking stage occurred at an informal dinner in October 1958 attended by himself, the Minister of Health, Dr. James McGrath, Miller and Dr. R.V. Christie, Professor of Medicine at McGill University.[3] Christie had come to Newfoundland as one of the speakers at the NMA annual fall refresher course and to conduct teaching rounds. He seems to have been impressed by the program provided for him and in conversation after dinner asked if any thought had been given to founding a medical school in Newfoundland.[3] McGrath and Miller both said the idea had never crossed their minds and certainly they did not expect to see it in their lifetimes. But Rusted was stimulated to set the wheels turning. If there was to be a Medical School, there would have to be a great deal of preliminary work gathering information, so that a brief could be prepared detailing the requirements and costs. During the next few years Rusted assembled the material required[4] and in September 1963 he wrote to the Minister of Health reviewing the present status of health services in the province.[5]

The key point in his letter to the Minister was his belief that "we ought to be actively considering a Medical School" for two reasons.[5] The supply of physicians from the British Isles, on which rural Newfoundland had been so dependent was beginning to diminish. Secondly, Dr. J.W. McLeod, the Executive Secretary of the Association of Canadian Medical Colleges(ACMC) had expressed the opinion that a second Medical School for the Atlantic provinces should be considered.

Rusted's suggestion was favourably received by the Minister but McGrath and Miller had their own concerns about medical manpower. The Children's Health Plan and and the Federal/Provincial Hospital Insurance plan had increased the demand for services in a province with far too few health professionals, a situation that could only worsen if, as expected, some form of universal health care was in the offing.

The Minister arranged for a meeting attended by himself, Miller and Rusted with representatives from Memorial University of

Newfoundland (MUN) and the NMA.[6] The group agreed with Rusted's suggestion and then asked MUN to extend an invitation to Dr. J. McLeod of the ACMC and Dr. C. Stewart, Dean of the Dalhousie University Medical School, to conduct a preliminary investigation on the feasibility of a medical school.[7]

In June 1964 the Royal Commission on Health Services released its report. It included a recommendation for a second medical school for the Atlantic provinces at Moncton or St. John's.[3] The Commission also recommended the establishment of a health resources fund (HRF) to provide the federal share of federal/provincial matched programs for the building of health facilities of national importance. One month later McLeod, on behalf of himself and Stewart, forwarded their report to the University.[8] They recommended a feasibility study in depth for a medical school. Furthermore, they suggested that the Medical School should be part of a "Health Sciences Centre" (HSC). This was a new concept involving the gathering together under one roof or in adjoining buildings all the facilities and resources required for undergraduate and postgraduate training of health professionals, and would have to include a university hospital and research laboratories. They enumerated the reasons why Newfoundland should actively pursue the establishment of a medical school. Besides those already cited they noted the beneficial effect of a medical school on health care generally in the province but, more significantly, Stewart warned that by 1970 Dalhousie University might not be able to accommodate its present number of Newfoundland applicants. The two signatories noted that the Royal Commission on Health Services had recommended a second medical school for the Atlantic provinces and in addition, through the HRF, the provision of financial resources towards its construction.

In May 1965 the President of the University acting on the McLeod/Stewart report appointed a joint advisory committee with representation from the NMA, MUN as well as Miller and McGrath under the chairmanship of Edgar House, a member of the board of Regents at MUN, to advise on implementation of the report.[3] The advisory committee recommended to the President that a commission be constituted to conduct a survey in depth of the feasibility of a medical school. The commission known as the MacFarlane commission, after its chairman Dr. J.A. MacFarlane, Dean Emeritus, Faculty of Medicine, University of Toronto, presented its report to President Gushue of MUN on 2 February 1966.[9] The commission endorsed the McLeod/Stewart recommendations for an HSC on campus to include a 400-bed University Hospital.

Upon receipt of the MacFarlane Commission report, the University constituted yet another committee with representation from the University, NMA, and the Department of Heath to advise the President on "the implications of the report and to advise on its implementation"[7] as well as to prepare a brief to Lord Brain who was delaying submitting his report until he had the opportunity to consider the University's brief for a medical school. Upon its receipt a few months later, Lord Brain came out in support of the MacFarlane Commission's recommendations.[3] With this backing the University moved on and appointed a planning committee with Dr. J.F. McCreary, President of the ACMC and Dean of the Faculty of Medicine, University of British Columbia, as chairman to carry the preparation of the brief for the medical school to its ultimate stage. The NMA and the Department of Health were not involved in this phase, but the NMA was kept in the picture.

On 6 September 1966 the planning committee submitted its report to the University, endorsing the MacFarlane Commission's report and recommending that steps be initiated to appoint a Dean. The Senate of the University gave its seal of approval to both these recommendations, subject to the Government's financial commitment to capital and operational costs and provided that the funding of the medical school did not come out of education grants to the University.

The Senate's endorsement of a medical school was officially presented to the Premier in November, 1966.[10] In the Speech from the Throne shortly afterwards, the government indicated its intention of establishing a " Medical College."[7] On 18 April 1967 Smallwood wrote to the University signifying the government's approval of the Senate resolution and noting that the government would have to provide forty to fifty million dollars in capital expenditures over the next five to six years.[11] This the government was willing to do, provided it received Federal support. The University took this as a green light to proceed. Dr. Ian Rusted was appointed

Dean as of 1 September 1967, recruitment of faculty began, and the first class was admitted in 1969. Presumably the University reasoned that the government would proceed quickly with an HSC, but in fact this did not happen because at this point the government began to have second thoughts about a medical school. The events leading to this change of heart began in September 1967 about the time McGrath was replaced by J.C. Crosbie as Minister of Health. Relations between Miller and the new Minister were never close.[12] Crosbie had his reservations about the ability of the province to support a medical school – concerns that were to become more vocal after he broke with Smallwood. The lack of rapport between Crosbie and Miller may have contributed to the subsequent vacillating conduct of the government towards it.

There is no record of Miller's opinion being sought before Smallwood made his written commitment to a medical school. But back in August 1965 the department had come out in favour of a medical school in its brief to the Brain Commission.[13] In principle, then, Miller must have supported the idea. Nevertheless he was a dispassionate man and in conversations with officials in his department showed that he realized that it might well have adverse consequences. Once it had provided the medical manpower for the province's needs, it would then become an exporter of physicians, he told Boyd Suttie, Assistant Deputy Minister of Health. Was that what the government wanted? He would have preferred arrangements with Dalhousie University to admit more Newfoundlanders and a continuation of student bursaries to meet medical manpower needs. Another physician related that Miller wondered if the operational costs would prove to be so heavy that the medical school would become an "albatross around the government's neck." Nevertheless, Miller seems to have considered the pros and cons carefully and concluded the benefits outweighed the drawbacks. Once he did so he never wavered in his backing. This in spite of the fact that he realized financial support of the medical school would come out of the Department of Health's budget. But he made it quite clear that this should not be at the expense of other programs of the department.

To understand the confusing events of the next few years it must be realized that the University was adamant in its commitment to a medical school but linked it to its taking the form of an HSC.[3] It refused to entertain the idea of the former without the latter. Better no medical school than one ill equipped for its task. Opposition to a medical school came from two quarters. There were those who, though appalled at the capital costs of an HSC, were willing to accept a medical school provided upgraded facilities of the St. John's hospitals were incorporated for clinical teaching and investigation in place of an HSC. Others, concerned at the operational costs of a medical school, rejected the whole idea out of hand. The question of an HSC was therefore irrelevant to their arguments. Some, such as Smallwood, oscillated between the two camps although no reference to second thoughts about the medical school appear in Smallwood's autobiography.*

For the government, the most pressing question was the funding of the HSC. The major portion would have to come out of the HRF. The formula for disbursement from this fund was complicated. Part was to be distributed on a nation-wide per capita basis, another part, especially earmarked for the Atlantic provinces, was also to be distributed on a per capita basis, and finally there was one hundred and seventy-five million dollars to be disbursed at the discretion of the federal Minister of NH&W. The problem was that Newfoundland's share from the first two sources would only come to about seventeen million six hundred thousand dollars, far short of the thirty million required to match the ten to twenty million dollars the province would be able to contribute. The shortfall could only be made up from the unalloted one hundred and seventy-five million dollars. The other provinces were unsympathetic to allowing Newoundland a special grant from this fund and wanted it divided on a nation-wide per capita basis. As a member of the advisory committee for disbursement of the HRF, Miller was well aware of these ripples.[15]

To add to the confusion, the Cabinet and the Department of Health had different ideas about the future of the General Hospital. The cabinet seems to have been under the impression that in the

* In his memoirs, all Smallwood had to say about the Medical School were these comments: "I brought out the great medical leader Lord Brain to advise us on the question of establishing a medical school. . .for a long time the only support I had for my proposal to start the medical college was Dr. Gordon Thomas, Chief of the Grenfell Hospital at St. Anthony."[14]

coming years, not only might it have to find funds for its share of the HSC but would also have to expend extensive sums in upgrading the General Hospital as an acute treatment centre. In those times of short money, the prospect was frightening. On the other hand, the Department of Health seems to have been quite clear, as far back as 1966, that the new University Hospital at the HSC would replace the General as an acute treatment facility. The buildings of the old General Hospital could then be converted into a chronic care and convalescent institution and also provide facilities for adult rehabilitation.[16]

But the most decisive event that pushed the provincial government to try and get out of its commitments to a medical school, was its deteriorating financial state. The post-war boom had ended and with it extravagant spending. There were fears that the province would not be able to meet present commitments without increased federal assistance.[17] Retrenchment was mandatory.[18] With such a bleak prospect in view, it was perhaps understandable that the government would want to liquidate an expensive commitment such as a medical school.

In December 1967 during a television interview Smallwood questioned the need for a University Hospital.[3] In reply, Rusted made it quite clear that University sponsorship of the medical school was a predicated on the construction of the HSC and that no renovations of the existing hospitals in St. John's could replace this need.[3] Smallwood took no further action.

There were other influences working against the medical school proposal. The NMA had always officially given its support, but there were individual physicians who were opposed. One of these, of some standing, had communicated his views privately to Smallwood in 1966.[19] Then in the summer of 1968 another influential physician sent a brief to the Department of Health listing reasons against a medical school.[20] The first physician associated himself with the opinions of the second.[19] The effect of these two communications on Smallwood was to undermine still further his commitment to a medical school. On the surface Smallwood appeared assured and opinionated, but in fact his self-confidence was easily shaken by the last person who spoke to him or the latest document he had read. After receiving these communications he appeared to

Rusted as not knowing what to do. "Whom am I to believe?"he is said to have exclaimed. M– and R– who give good reasons for not going ahead with a Medical School or you who give good reasons for having one. What am I to do?"

At the instruction of Smallwood, copies of the brief and the supporting letters from the two physicians, were circulated to the NMA and to the University for their comments. The executive committee of the NMA must have been embarrassed by the actions of two of its members acting on their own responsibility. It reiterated its support of the medical school unless new evidence showed that "it was no longer fiscally practical."[21] The university in its reply threw its support behind the NMA's response and then proceeded to question the arguments in the opposing brief.[22]

About this time Dr. C. Stewart, the Dean of Medicine at Dalhousie University, in the course of a convocation address, happened to mention that there had been a drop in the number of qualified applicants from Newfoundland for admission to the medical school.[23] In the previous years the number had been increasing rapidly. The Dean speculated that if this trend continued Dalhousie might be able to admit all properly qualified Newfoundland applicants. It will be recalled that one of the arguments for a second medical school in the Atlantic Provinces was the possibility that Dalhousie University might find it could not admit sufficient numbers of properly qualified Newfoundland applicants. Dr. Stewart, when clarification of his remarks was sought by the NMA replied: " I would not wish to give anyone the impression I am opposing the development of another medical school in the Atlantic provinces."[23] He added that his support of a medical school in 1964 had been predicated upon an anticipated continued marked increase in the number of applications for admission from Newfoundland. But in fact this trend had stopped. His less than lukewarm support for a new medical school in the Atlantic provinces only added to peoples' hesitations.

The government may have procrastinated but not Miller, who meanwhile had the task of budgeting for the medical school. He argued that the school could be regarded as a project of national importance and therefore entitled for special consideration and extra funds from the HRF.[24] He warned the Minister that in the present climate of government indecision and with the medical school proceeding with recruitment " [we] are getting . . . more deeply involved every day." He told the Minister that "from the point of view of pure economics there was no case for a Medical School in Newfoundland," but then listed the well-known benefits. A few months later Miller reminded the Minister that the government had yet to allocate its share of capital costs for the HSC.[25] Subsequently he was asked to comment on the opposing brief of the influential physician.[20] He went through it point by point questioning the validity of its claims and deductions.[26] He concluded with the warning that, at the request of the government, "in good faith Memorial University had agreed to undertake what they described as this tremendous task. If there is a change of policy at this time the repercussions on the University and Hospital and Medical Services and indeed on the government will be immeasurable . . . However if there is a possibility of a change in policy it should be announced at an early date so that the disappointment and other adverse effects will not continue to multiply." In other words, the government had made a commitment and should stick to it. He used to say privately that in the history of Newfoundland nothing had been investigated as thoroughly as the question of a Medical School.

Still the government continued to drag its feet. Miller wrote to the Minister stating that he had raised the question of Newfoundland's "getting something from the unallotted portion of the HRF, but had got no support."[27] Consequently he had "suggested to Rusted that between us, we should prepare a comprehensive brief for Munroe" [The Federal Minister of NH&W]. Rusted warned the government that unless it moved quickly it might not be able to obtain the full thirty million dollars it needed from the HRF.[3] Finally, in January 1971, the government adopted the plan of replacing the General Hospital by a University Hospital and transforming the former into a chronic care institute. It applied for and received the thirty million dollars from the HRF and construction of the HSC commenced.[28]

It seems surprising that it took five years for the cabinet to come around to the obvious solution mentioned by Boyd Suttie to Miller in 1966 and proposed by others since that date.

Chapter 12 – Notes

1. MacLeod, Malcolm *A Bridge Built Halfway. A history of Memorial College,* 1925-50 McGill-Queen's University Press, Montreal & Kingston 1990 p. 235.

2. *The Medical School* (Editorial) Newfoundland Medical Association Newsletter 8 (6): 5.1966.

3. Rusted, I.E. Faculty of Medicine Memorial University of Newfoundland. In: *New Medical Schools at Home and Abroad,* edited by John Z. Bowers and Elizabeth F. Purcell, Josiah Macey Foundation Independent Publishing Group 14 Vanderventer Ave. Port Washington, N.Y. 11050 1978.

4. Rusted, I.E. *The Case for A Medical School in Newfoundland.* Newfoundland Medical Association Newsletter 6 (4): 812 1964.

5. CNS IRC IR to JMcG 1963-09-06.

6. ANLMA IR Address to Newfoundland Medical Association 1968-06-07.

7. CNS EMRC Morgan, M.O. Address to the Doctors attending the annual fall refresher course 1968-10-24.

8. ANLMA. J.W. McL to RG 1964 -08-24.

9. CNS JRSC Publicity Release by Memorial University of Newfoundland. 1966-02-15.

10. CNS JRSC MOM to JRS 1966- 11-2.

11. CNS JRSC JRS to MOM 1967-04-18.

12. NRC Miller, L.A. Memoir, unpublished.

13. PANL PRC 19 Health Box 35-1-6-1. Brief by Department of Health to the Royal Commission on Health. 1965- 08 -19.

14. Smallwood JR ibid. p. 386.

15. CNS EMRC LAM Memo 1966-07-20.

16. CNS JCCC BS to LAM 1966-03-9.

17. CNS JCCC JCCtoJRS 1968-04-16.

18. CNS EMRC ER Memo to Ex Council 1969-02-04.

19. ANLMA JBR to JRS 1968-08-28.

20. ANLMA ARM Brief to Department of Health (undated).

21. ANLMA PJW to TAH 1968-9-18.

22. ANLMA MOM to TAH 1968-10-4 .

23. ANLMA CBS to WDP 1968-10-18.

24. CNSJCCC LAM to JCC 1968-01-16.

25. CNS JCCC LAM to JCC 1968-04-08.

26. CNS EMRC LAM to TAH 1968-08 -19 .

27. CNS EMRC LAM to ER 1969-5-16.

28. CNS JRSC ER Memo to Ex Council 1971 01 08.

CHAPTER 13

The International Grenfell Association

To appreciate relations between the government and the IGA in Miller's day, one has to compare them with those in previous years and after his retirement.*

Medical services in the Northern reaches of Newfoundland developed independently of those of the south. They owe their origins to Dr., later Sir Wilfred Grenfell. In 1892 he was sent out from the UK, as a medical missionary, by the National Mission to Deep-sea Fishermen** (RNMDSF) to the Newfoundland fishermen who migrated each year to fish off the coasts of Labrador. Many brought their families which they would house in make-shift settlements on the coast. In the autumn they would return to their homes on the Island. There were also a few permanent fishing settlements on the Labrador coast. Grenfell was appalled by the abject poverty he encountered among the fishermen and their families. He came to the conclusion that it was not enough to minister to their medical and spiritual needs, but he would also have to try to better their social and economic circumstances. Over the years under his dynamic, vigorous but somewhat erratic leadership, a network of community nursing stations, hospitals, schools, orphanages, craftshops and cooperative stores were erected along the coast of Labrador and the tip of the Northern Peninsula. This multifaceted corporation came to

* I am indebted to *Grenfell of Labrador, A Biography* by R. Rompkey for much of this chapter.

**It acquired the prefex Royal in 1897.

be world renowned and held up as a model for providing comprehensive social services in remote areas. But it was Grenfell's business ventures that landed him in hot water. The merchants of St. John's were generous in their support of his missionary and medical activities, but resented his intrusion into their business affairs.

By 1913 the transatlantic operations of the RNMDSF had grown so large that by mutual consent they were incorporated into a separate organization, known as the International Grenfell Association (IGA).

Grenfell soon found that his talents were those of a promoter and circuit lecturer rather than a physician. He was a charismatic figure able to hold audiences spellbound with descriptions of the wilds of Labrador and the hardship of life there. More importantly, his listeners responded by reaching into their pockets.

Grenfell's speaking and fund-raising engagements were spectacularly successful and from his mid-forties most of his time was spent criss-crossing North America and the UK, promoting his mission and leaving the medical services in the competent hands of Dr. J.M. Little and later Drs. C.S . Curtis and H.L. Paddon.[1] As a result of his strenuous lecture tours he built up a large endowment fund for the IGA.

But Grenfell didn't stop there. A steady stream of books poured forth from his pen, publicizing his achievements and adventures. They came to occupy a high rank in the inspirational literature of the day, the sort of book one gave to a favourite nephew with the hope that it might prod him into doing something with his life.

No wonder that by the 1920s "the Grenfell Mission" was a household word throughout the English speaking world.

There was however, another side to all these promotional activities. To persuade people to donate to the IGA, Grenfell had to paint Labrador in lurid colors. This did not sit well with the authorities in St. John's. They accused Grenfell of exaggeration, giving a false picture of the place in the eyes of the world and frightening off investors. Grenfell in turn accused them of callousness and incompetence. These accusations and counter accusations hardly made for a harmonious partnership.

The government's attitude towards the IGA, at the best, could be described as ambivalent. Because of the IGA's and Grenfell's world-wide reputation it had to be handled with care. The government was also grateful to be relieved of responsibility for providing health care in the northern parts of the colony. In recognition of the IGA's role as a provider of health care, the government, with some misgivings,* began to give it an annual grant-in-aid which by 1932 was fifteen thousand dollars. In that year, because of hard times, it was forced to stop payments.[2]

Relations did not improve under the Commission of Government. It was in the welfare functions of the Department of PH &W that friction occurred. The IGA's repeated failure, in spite of warnings, to provide proper accounting for disbursement of welfare funds, was a source of intense irritation to Puddester and Mosdell.[3]

Grenfell's personality quirks only added fuel to the flames. He was a law unto himself and took no pains to conceal his opinions of people he disliked. Relations must have reached an all time low when Puddester sent this blistering letter to Grenfell: "[You have denounced me] as a politician first and all the time and an incompetent one at that, unfit to run the department over which I have been called by the UK government to preside . . . when you did have occasion to communicate about health and welfare matters from 1930 to 1932, it was always over my head as the one in charge of these matters as secretary of state."[4]

Another cause of resentment was the size of the annual grant-in-aid which had been reinstated by the new regime, but only at two thousand five hundred dollars. A request for an increase was met with the answer that the privilege of importing goods without paying duty was in itself the equivalent of a grant.[5] Eventually, an agreement was reached by which the IGA would pay duty on imported goods and in return the government would give it a rebate equivalent to the duties it paid.[6] The government would also continue the annual grant-in-aid then set at two thousand five hundred dollars.

In 1937, Grenfell retired as superintendent of the IGA to be succeeded by Dr. C.S. Curtis, an easier person to work with. But Grenfell's departure also spelled the end of the steady flow of money into the IGA coffers. His successor did not have his matchless fund-raising talents. As the years passed the IGA began to experience increasing difficulties

* For fear that if the government subsidized one charity, others would ask for the same privilege.

matching expenses with the revenue from the interest on its endowments, forcing it to turn increasingly to the government for assistance.[7] This marked the beginning of the loss of its independence. It was also about this time that Miller became Deputy Minister.

One reason for the mission's growing financial troubles was paradoxically the increasing prosperity of the communities it serviced, firstly following Confederation and then the construction of the Pinetree extension bases of the DEW* line by the Americans in the early 1950s. The result was an escalation of wages and costs.[8] In 1952 Dr. C.S. Curtis, superintendent of the Mission, wrote to Miller that even with the help it was receiving the IGA was finding it difficult to meet its commitments.[9] The choices were either to increase the fees the Mission tried to collect for its services or turn over its health facilities and programs to the government. He gloomily wondered, "... perhaps the days of this Mission are over. I do not know the answer. [I am writing to you] because you are sympathetic to the Mission." As an aside he made the comment that he doubted that the government could provide the same services as cheaply. These were exactly the sentiments of the Department of Health.[10]

Miller's philosophy was that he had enough worries running the Health Services in the other parts of the province and was delighted to have the IGA relieve him of the burden at the top of the Northern Peninsula and Labrador. He never interfered in its internal operations and was unwavering in its support. Relations during his day between the government and the IGA were always cordial, perhaps in part because Health and Welfare were now separate departments. It was only after his retirement that "cracks began to appear in what had been a happy association."[8] Still, as the years passed during Miller's term, the Mission became increasingly dependent on the government for its operational costs.[10, 11] The IGA also looked to the government for capital expenditures incurred in renovations and in the building of nursing stations and hospitals.[12] This did not stop the IGA from extending its commitments. With the blessing of the government, the IGA contracted with BRINCO** to provide Health Services to Churchill Falls in Labrador during and after the construction of the hydro-electric power plant and dam.

* Distant Early Warning

** British Newfoundland Corporation

The Department reaped benefits from its partnership with IGA. The IGA had large endowments and the interest from these was used to provide services which otherwise would not have existed or for which the government would have had to find the funds itself.

G.W. Thomas, the Chief Surgeon of the Mission and its Superintendent after 1964, came to know Miller intimately and the two men developed a close and warm relationship. After Miller had told Thomas to drop in whenever he was in St. John's, many were the dinners and luncheons they had together at the Miller house. Thomas's recollections provide a picture of how Miller appeared to those who worked with him, and why he was so greatly respected by those who came into contact with him:

> He was a quiet man. A man of few words. You could talk to him freely and know he would not betray a confidence. He was also a man of his word. If he said he would do something, you didn't need it in writing. He was extremely business-like. He would go over a proposal item by item registering approval or disagreement. He was particularly good at working out the financial costs and hazarding a guess about whether there might or might not be funds available for a project. As you were talking to him you felt he was sizing you up, but you didn't feel at all threatened. His judgements of people were astute. He was an ideal civil servant of the old type, never disloyal to government, although obviously sometimes he was extremely frustrated. He had a tremendous compassion for Newfoundland. For him his work was not just a job, but a way of serving his country. After he retired, he joined the Board of the IGA. He was tremendously valuable because he knew how governments worked.

Patricia Thomas, Gordon's wife, remembers his many visits to St. Anthony, usually just before bad weather. If Miller was coming, so was the fog. He usually stayed at the Thomases' home. The first visit stands out in her memory. The morning after his arrival

> he came down in his slippers after my husband had gone to work. He chatted over breakfast. He asked me many questions about my hopes and plans for the future, my interest in my husband's work. It was only years later that he told me he

always followed the same procedure; whenever he visited a Cottage Hospital he cornered the wife as soon as possible to find out if she was happy; if she was, then it was likely the couple would stay; if she was discontented it was a waste of time to discuss future plans with the husband.

Miller seems to have had great confidence in Thomas. Once in his early days, Miller telegraphed him to go and see a patient suffering from a stroke in Jackson's Arm, well outside the IGA territory. Thomas had a harrowing walk of 18 miles over snow and ice to the patient's home. On his return, Thomas telephoned Miller to report the results of his trip. He was curious that Miller had asked him to undertake this arduous trip. Miller replied "I felt that you, but no other doctor would do it ."

Similar stories are told by other physicians of Miller's concern that a patient in the most isolated of spots was not overlooked. Of course he also saw that the physician was rewarded for his pains!

Miller would choose someone in whom he had confidence to go as his deputy or troubleshooter to investigate a situation that was causing the department concern. On one occasion he sent Thomas to conduct clinics at a health centre that was in trouble, just outside the IGA area, and to report his findings and recommendations for correcting its problems.

Miller's support of the IGA went beyond passive non-intervention. He was tireless in finding government money for IGA's research and programs for its extensive and successful campaign to eradicate tuberculosis. Through his friendship with Percy E. Moore, Superintendent of Medical Services Federal Indian Affairs Bureau, Miller obtained support for the anti-TB program amongst the native peoples of Labrador.

The events surrounding the building of the Charles S. Curtis Hospital were a test of the strength of Miller's and Thomas's friendship. In 1962, at the request of Dr. Charles S. Curtis, the former superintendent of the IGA, a delegation of the Board of Directors of the IGA conducted an assessment of the Mission's health facilities. It labelled the hospital at St. Anthony as "messy, overcrowded and badly in need of improvement."[13] Smallwood had given Thomas his unlisted telephone number and had told him to call him directly whenever he wanted. This was one of the occasions when Thomas took him at his word. He arranged an appointment with Smallwood and flew to St. John's. He told Smallwood that "the [St. Anthony] Hospital is cramped, outdated and must be rebuilt."[14] But the mere rebuilding of the St. Anthony Hospital was not what Thomas had in mind. The time had now come for something more ambitious. Expanding industrial development in Labrador and Northern Newfoundland justified he believed a 250 (later reduced to 170) bed hospital that would serve as the regional hospital and referral center for the IGA territory and provide also basic speciality care. With a medical school probably in the offing, Thomas hoped that the Mission's resources would be used for teaching and training in what has come to be called circumpolar health, i.e. the diseases and health services peculiar to frigid regions. Consequently, the new hospital should be equipped to accommodate and teach medical students and residents. Smallwood agreed in principal with Thomas's request and then called Miller and instructed him and Thomas to get in touch with the Department of Public Works to start work on planning and constructing the new hospital. Thomas recalls that while Miller must have been annoyed at being by-passed and, as so often happened, Smallwood's not consulting the Department of Health before agreeing to the new hospital, he appears never to have borne Thomas any ill will. Relations were just as cordial afterwards as before.

From the mid-century onwards the IGA began to experience a rising tide of criticisms. As the government increasingly became the paymaster, the relevance of the IGA began to be questioned. Furthermore, like the cottage hospital scheme, it was accused of paternalism and stifling local initiative. But none of these criticisms were allowed to change the harmonious relations between the IGA and the government in the Smallwood era. It was only later that these rumblings of discontent came to a head, ending in 1978 with the IGA turning over its health services, but not its endowments, to the Government of Newfoundland.

Chapter 13 – Notes

1. Thomas G. *Grenfell, Little, Curtis and Paddon*. Newfoundland Medical Association Newsletter. 16: 16-20 1974.

2. PANL GN 38 S6-1-1 EABW to JCP 1935-04-01.

3. PANL GN 38 S6-1-1 HM to JCP 1934-09-21.

4. PANL GN 38 S6-1-1 JCP to WTG 1935-08-28.

5. PANL GN 38 S6-5-1 Com. of G with IGA reps 1935-06-25.

6. PANL GN 38 S6-5-1 Com. of G with IGA reps 1935-06-29.

7. CNS JRSC PSF Memo to Ex Council 1954-03-22.

8. Thomas G. Personal Communication.

9. CNS JRSC CSC to LAM 1952-09-18.

10. CNS JRSC JMcG Memo 1957-03-27.

11. Thomas, Gordon W. *From Sled to Satellite–My Years in the Grenfell Mission*, Irwin Publishing Inc., Toronto . Printed in Canada by John Deyell Co. 1987

12. CNS JRSC J. McG Memo 1962-01-29.

13. Thomas G. ibid. p.84.

14. Thomas G. ibid. p. 85.

CHAPTER 14

The Government Hospitals in St. John's

In Miller's day the government owned and operated three hospitals in St. John's: The General Hospital, The Sanatorium and the Hospital for Mental and Nervous Diseases (now the Waterford Hospital). The General occupied most of Miller's attention because it was the only one to have an MAC of which Miller became Chairman, *ex officio*, when the St. John's Government Hospitals were added to his responsibilities as DMS.[1*]

The General Hospital had been a Military Hospital until 1870, but on withdrawal of the British garrison had been taken over by the government and run as an acute care civilian hospital, an unusual action for a government to take in North America in those days.[2] Until after World War I, it was the only hospital in St. John's. When Miller became DMS in 1944 it had 165 beds.[3] In the 1920s it had a Board of Governors, but this had disappeared by the time Miller was appointed DMS. During the days of Commission of Government, government hospitals were run directly by the Department of PH&W. In his earlier days as chairman of the MAC of the General Hospital, Miller is described as "arrogant, arbitrary, and deciding on his own responsibility which recommendations of the MAC to take to the Commission Government and summarily refusing to pass on others. However, he quickly learned to change his tune and soon settled down and became more circumspect".[4]

* It is not recorded when this happened. Perhaps after Sir John Puddester's death.

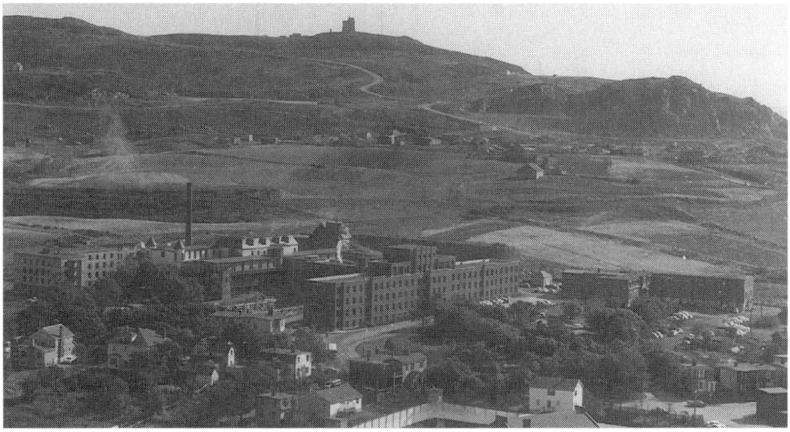

The General Hospital St. John's, circa 1950 ***Centre:*** *Puddester Wing;* ***Rear:*** *Old wards and Military Hospital;* ***Right:*** *Fever Hospital*
Courtesy Lillian Stevenson, Nursing Archives Museum.

St. John's grew rapidly after 1949, tripling its population in a quarter of a century. The General and the two private hospitals (St. Clare's and the Grace General) expanded to keep pace with the city's growth and prosperity and by 1959 the General had grown to 446 beds.[5] The years after the war also saw an influx of young Newfoundland doctors returning with specialist qualifications.

In those days (before accreditation forced hospitals to limit admitting privileges to one hospital per doctor) returning specialists were appointed to the staff of all three St. John's hospitals;but the General, as the largest and the sole referral centre for the Cottage Hospitals, was where they looked for most of their patients. Inevitably, conflicts broke out between the impatient young specialists, "young Turks" they called themselves, who were pushing for changes with the old guard physicians who were quite content with things as they were. Many of these disputes were fought out at the MAC. There were two perennial sources of dispute. The first was the resistance of the older physicians to sharing their quotas of patient beds with the younger ones. The second was the ridiculously low fees for treating referrals from the Cottage Hospitals, a schedule that had not changed since 1936.

One colleague remembers Miller presiding at the head of the table. "He said little, never pushed his views and never got involved

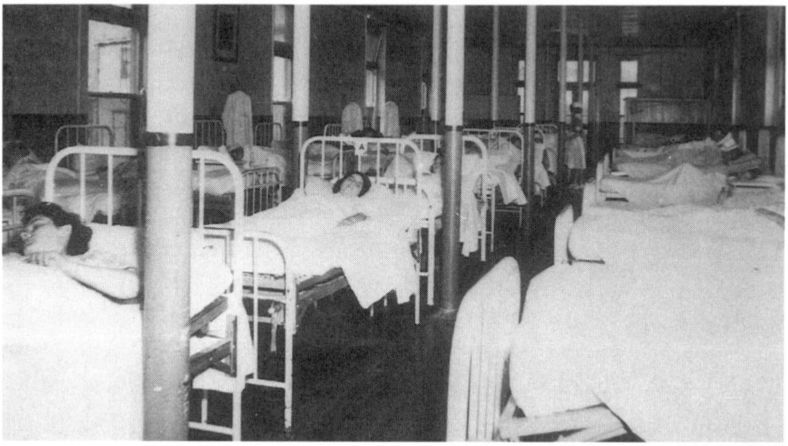

General Hospital, Cowan Ward circa 1940
Courtesy Lillian Stevenson, Nursing Archives Museum

in controversy. If a project involving expenditure of money came up, he said "he would see what he could do." To a less friendly member of the Council, he appeared for all the world like a "Buddha – plump, bland and complacent."

Two entirely different pictures of Miller's administration of the General Hospital have come down. To one member of the MAC, he appeared "staid and conservative, he just didn't want to move. He wasn't in the least way progressive. Perhaps he couldn't buck the old guard who didn't want to entertain any competition. They blocked everything". He could never understand the admiration for Miller. "When you went to see him, he said almost nothing. Perhaps that is why people thought him so wise. To me, his mind appeared pedestrian compared to McGrath's [The Minister of Health], who was brilliant." The same critic recalls an incipient staff revolt when each of the malcontents was ordered by the Minister of Health to put his signature at the end of a blank piece of paper above which the Minister said he would write a new set of by-laws for the hospital. "We all caved in because we were afraid of losing our jobs."

On the other hand Miller's admirers point to the achievements of the years after World War II. A new wing was built in 1945 and in 1960 and 1961 there were further extensions. Even so, there was always a shortage of beds. It is true renovations were always slow in coming, but this was not Miller's fault. It was beyond his control because construction and maintenance came under the Department of Public Works and had to be paid for out of its budget. Public Works was as short of funds as the Department of Health and getting it to undertake renovations required monumental persistence and persuasion. For years, in spite of complaints from the Department of Health, outpatients faced an unsightly view of rows of uncovered pipes in the ceiling because Public Works insisted plumbers must have ready access to them. However when it came to purchasing new equipment and establishing coronary and intensive care units, the General was not slow compared to other hospitals. A coronary care unit was established as early as 1967.

Which impression of Miller is right? Was he an obstacle to progress or was he an energetic reforming administrator? The answer is neither. Miller was never a crusader for some pet project. It was a waste of time to get into an argument with him. He wouldn't budge. It was useless to expect him to push aside the entrenched old guard. It was unreasonable to expect him to commit political suicide by engaging in head-on collisions. Miller was not a creative thinker, he did not come up with new schemes. His mind did not work that way. But he was a great listener to the ideas of others and could recognize those that had merit and, above all, those that were workable. He had an open mind and could be persuaded to adopt new schemes. Those with the art of persuasion and who could convince him of the wisdom of a certain course of action, could then count on his steady support and tireless efforts to find funds for its implementation. Thus Dr. Ian Rusted was able to persuade him to provide space and funds for a radioactive iodine laboratory.

Miller was tremendously proud of the General Hospital and made it his aim to see that it was as up to date as any on the Mainland. Up to the time of Medicare he jealously guarded its position as the sole referral centre for the Cottage Hospitals against attempts by the private hospitals to encroach on its preserve. In his eyes it was "the flagship of the government-owned fleet of hospitals," recalls a physician of those times . He would come on a tour of inspection every six months but more frequently during building periods. A quizzical streak would surface at these times, according to one who remembers accompanying him on these tours. "He would always go to a particular corner to see if a speck of dust present on his previous visit had been removed. He would then return to tell me triumphantly that it hadn't, but he would never tell me where it was."[6] This ritual went on for several years.

Miller realized that a lever for winning approval for improvements was accreditation. Accreditation of hospitals goes back to the 1920s when the American College of Surgeons started to accredit hospitals in the USA and later in Canada. After World War II accreditation in Canada was taken over by the Canadian Council of Hospital Accreditation, and soon no hospital could afford to be without it. Miller was quick to use recommendations of the accreditators as a means for forcing changes while the ruinous consequences of withdrawal of accreditation was a weapon he could hold over the government's head. The General Hospital was accredited by 1948[7] and possibly had been as far back as the 1920s. During Miller's career it was always fully accreditated except in his last few years when it was given provisional accreditation until a Board of Directors had been appointed.

Miller also recognized that being accredited as a teaching hospital was another way of bringing pressure to bear for needed changes. While away pursuing post graduate studies, Dr. Ian Rusted had written to Miller in 1949 indicating his interest in working for the General Hospital to obtain recognition for it as a post graduate training centre.[8] Miller saw that he was given the opportunity to do so, which he did with success.

As the years went by the anomaly of Miller being both the Deputy Minister and Chairman of the MAC at the General Hospital came under increasing fire. His positions allowed him to deal with an issue at two administrative levels which led to accusations of deviousness. He was also in a position that could put him in a conflict of interest. The chairman of the MAC should be an advocate of the hospital's interests which on occasion might not coincide with those of government. Miller's double administrative roles also undermined the position of the superintendent of the hospital. Staff often found it more advantageous to by-pass him and go directly to Miller. Miller never took the advice to resign from the position of Chairman of the MAC . He seems not to have appreciated the embarassing position in which he was putting the Superintendent.

The government hospital in St. John's with the most beds was the Hospital for Mental and Nervous Diseases (the Waterford).

For much of Miller's earlier years it was an eyesore: run down, overcrowded buildings and inadequate staff both in numbers and in training.[9] Before the era of psychopharmacy it was mainly a custodial institution. At the end of the war, Dr. C. Roberts became Superintendent and introduced radical changes in staffing and policies which led to improvements in patient care.[9, 10] Miller warned the government that several wings were fire hazards and needed to be replaced, but the Commission of Government, knowing its days were numbered, preferred not to undertake long-term commitments.[8] It was only in 1953, thanks to the federal NHGP, that these renovations were carried out.

Miller appears to have given less attention to the Hospital for Mental and Nervous Diseases than to the other areas of his responsibilities, perhaps because it was in capable hands and because there was no MAC to be managed. He didn't visit the hospital until Roberts asked him to do so. Miller demurred, before agreeing, saying that he did not wish to appear as if he were checking on him.[11] There was probably another unstated reason. Miller, having played the game himself, was well aware that his official visits could be used to confront him with obvious deficiencies and pointblank demands for immediate commitments to remedy them. He usually took care not to be trapped.

But if Miller felt he didn't have to worry about the administration of the Hospital for Mental and Nervous Diseases, the placement of deranged patients was quite another matter. Many are the stories of his being threatened by a frantic doctor to arrange admission for a demented patient or accept responsibility for the consequences. A physician in a remote locality telegraphed Miller requesting permission to admit a deranged woman, the wife of a distraught husband and mother of a household of naked, starving children, only to receive the standard reply that there were no beds. He wired back asking Miller's permission to request the RCMP to shoot the woman.[12] An air ambulance arrived the next day to take the patient to St. John's. On another occasion Miller had wired the father of a disturbed patient that there were no beds available. A few days later he received a telegram: ARRIVING ON THE NORTHERN RANGER WITH MY SON AND BRINGING A BED.

Chapter 14 – Notes

1. PANL Health and Public Welfare Act 1931, Acts of the General Assembly of Newfoundland.

2. Rusted, N. *The St. John's General Hospital. Historical and Personal.* Newfoundland Medical Association Newsletter 16 (3): 5 - 10 1975.

3. WDPC Vanderlehr R.A, Heering R.E *Report of a survey on civic health services as they relate to the health of Armed Forces in Newfoundland.* United States Public Health Service 3 December 1940. Unpublished.

4. Rusted, N. Personal Communication.

5. Miller, L. *The Newfoundland Department of Health.* Canadian Journal of Public Health 50 (6): 228-39, 1959.

6. Story, J. Personal Communication.

7. PANL GN 26/4.

8. Rusted, I.E. *Recollections of Continuing Medical Education in Newfoundland and Labrador.* Newfoundland Medical Association Newsletter 18 (1): 5-10. 1976

9. O'Brien, Patricia. *Out of Sight. A History of the Waterford Hospital.* Breakwater Books, St. John's, Newfoundland. AlC 6E6 1989.

10. Roberts, C.A. *From Fishing Cove to Faculty Council.* Pondhead Publisher Calgary, Alberta 1995.

11. Roberts CA ibid P. 56.

12. Thomas G. Personal Communication.

CHAPTER 15

The Cottage Hospital Scheme

In the memories of a host of physicians coming to Newfoundland from the British Isles, the Cottage Hospitals are indelibly associated with Leonard Miller. He was the one who had recruited them, and he was the one they would telephone upon arrival. Miller's children remember many an evening interrupted by a telephone call from a new arrival, often followed by his appearance soon after on their doorstep. Miller was sympathetic to their homesickness and trepidation at facing they knew not what on some remote windswept, bleak promontory. He was only too pleased to welcome them to his home and to calm their fears. Miller would also be the one they would remember and talk about years later when, as did so many, they moved to greener pastures.

Provision of health care in the remoter parts of Newfoundland has always been beset with shortages of staff. In the days before Commission of Government few outports could support a resident physician, and then often only intermittently. Not many physicians were willing to run the risks of such an uncertain livelihood. Those that were brave enough to settle in the outports frequently had to move when times got bad, and indeed the number of physicians in the outports was less in 1930 than in 1911.[1] Many operated on what was known as "the book system" whereby each family or single adult paid an annual fee which insured them for all medical services for the ensuing year.

In the 1920s, the Newfoundland Outport Nursing Industrial Association (NONIA), a voluntary organization, was founded to place district nurses in remote areas where there were no physicians.[2] This was progress, but by 1934 the numbers had shrunk to only 6 or 7 nurses.[2] Obviously the only way to attract and keep physicians in the outports would be to provide them with a salary. This was the rationale for the Cottage Hospital Scheme, as it was officially called.

Miller was wont to say, "I had very little to do with thinking up the idea of the Cottage Hospitals."[3] He then goes on "to put the credit where it belongs" by naming Sir John C. Puddester, and Dr. H. M. Mosdell.[4] In fact the idea was not new to Newfoundland.

Until the mid-nineteenth century hospitals were charitable institutions for the care of sick paupers. There was little that could be done in the way of active treatment. The discovery of anesthetics which revolutionized surgery and the development of good nursing care, changed the sceptical attitude towards hospitals. These activities could best be carried out in professionally staffed and properly equipped institutions. In rural areas, cottage hospitals were the answer.

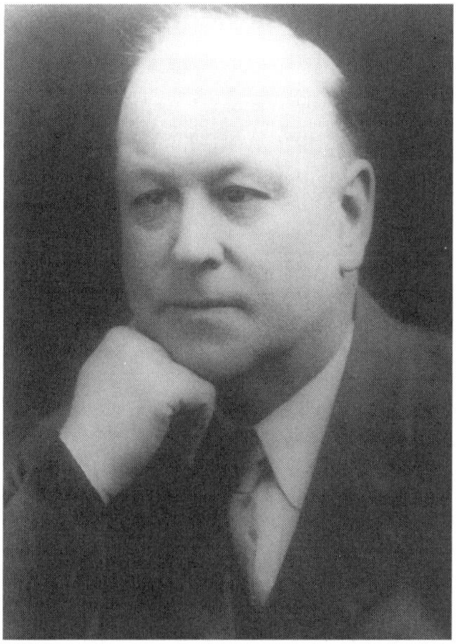

Sir John Puddester
Courtesy of Mr. Justice J. Puddester

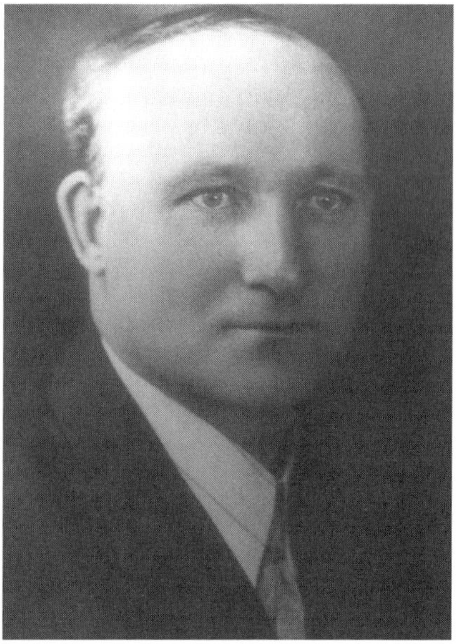

Dr. H.M. Mosdell
Courtesy Dr. R. Cooper

In the UK, the first was opened in 1859.[5] Their obvious benefits were soon widely appreciated and they multiplied rapidly. A controversial feature was the method of funding - payment of a weekly fee by subscribers entitling them to admission when needed.[5]

The first cottage hospital in Newfoundland, and a somewhat primitive one at that, was built in 1893 at Battle Harbour, Labrador, for Dr. Wilfred Grenfell.[3] He then went on to establish a much better equipped one at St. Anthony in 1899-1900, one which attracted patients from all over the island.[6] Through the tireless promotion of his mission, he spurred the demand for cottage hospitals in the colony so effectively, that in 1909 Sir Edward Morris included them in his election platform and won.[7]

Morris never implemented his promise, but this did not stop the construction of several small hospitals on the island through local or company initiatives.*

The idea of government-operated cottage hospitals lay dormant until 1930 when the Royal Commission on Health and Public Charities recommended their construction.[8] Strangely the Royal Commission made no reference to the model it already had at hand in the International Grenfell Association (IGA) network of community nursing stations staffed by nurse mid-wives linked to one large

* At Twillingate, Grand Falls and Grand Bank.

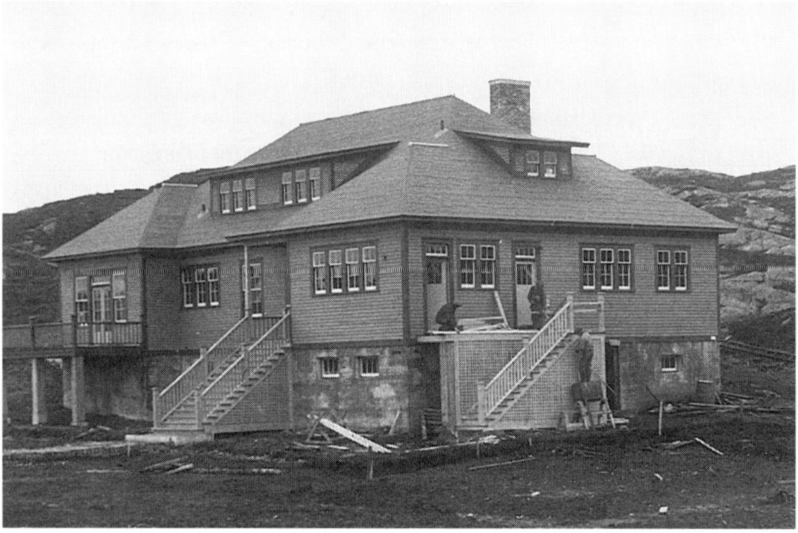

Burgeo Cottage Hospital *Courtesy Dr. Nigel Rusted*

cottage hospital (St. Anthony) and two smaller ones. Instead the commissioners referred glowingly to the physician-staffed cottage hospitals in the Highlands of Scotland and held these up as the pattern Newfoundland should emulate.

This was what the Commission of Government now proposed to do. With the benefit of hindsight we can see that it might have been wiser to have paid more heed to the experience of the IGA and less to the Highlands of Scotland; to have placed more emphasis on community nursing stations and less on physician-staffed cottage hospitals. However as Miller pointed out, the IGA had an excellent communications system which the Commission of Government lacked.[3] He was well aware of the arguments for and against the two philosophies for the provision of health care in remote areas and once said: "I think in some areas a good district nurse with a knowledge of the fundamentals of public health, provided she is in communication with the doctor can do just as much for the population as a doctor can, and the doctor, if he is in one of these small places only becomes frustrated anyway."[3]

How the department of PH&W envisaged the scheme should function, was laid out in a departmental memorandum prepared during the planning phase.[9] It was to be based on a partnership between the government as provider and the community as user – each with its entitlements and obligations. The government would assume the costs of the construction and operations of each hospital and reserved to itself the right of choice of location. If crown land was not available then the community would have to provide a site of at least four acres satisfactory to the government. Every able bodied adult male was expected to contribute voluntary labour to the extent that he was able. Each family would be required to pay an annual premium of four dollars for hospital and nursing services and two-fifty in regions where there was only a district medical officer. Able bodied adults unable to pay the premium would have to contribute "labour or in kind". Each settlement in a cottage hospital region was to have a committee of not more than three persons responsible for raising the premiums and settling who could not pay or who must pay in "labour or in kind." The settlement committees would report to the central or executive committee for their cottage hospital region. The central committee would comprise one delegate from each settlement committee and would be charged with the task of arranging collections in kind, the supervision of cash contributions towards the support of the hospital and the organization of free labour for the maintenance of the hospital.

The scheme as implemented seems to have differed in a number of respects from this blueprint and in fact local circumstances and changing times brought in still more modifications. In 1936 the family premium was set at five dollars per annum but over the years it gradually rose to fifteen dollars and somewhat higher in large centres (a single adult paid half the family premium).[4] There were extra charges for some services such as deliveries and dental extractions.[4] Local boards of health were appointed but proved to be a disappointment.* They were accused of intruding into the management of the cottage hospitals and dictating to the doctors. But whatever the reasons, they dwindled in importance and eventually disappeared, their fund-raising role being taken over by the secretary-treasurer or business managers of the cottage hospitals who came to wield considerable power.[4] Other components of the preliminary draft relating to free labour seemed to have been implimented only sporadically.[3]

What may seem surprising with so many struggling communities is the fact that 75–85% of those liable to pay premiums did so.[4,10] Among the defaulters it was a common practice to pay the premium when services were required.[11] Because of the high collection rate, as late as 1953, the government was able to fund 40% of the operating costs of the scheme from the premiums it collected.[12]

Construction of the first Cottage Hospitals began in 1935 and the last of the fourteen was opened in 1952.** Ownership and maintenance were vested in the Department of Public Works. There was no master plan for placing them.[3] Rarely, a Cottage Hospital was built in response to a petition from a region, but more often it was a government decision. There were occasions when the location was dictated by blatantly political considerations such as at Old Perlican in Puddester's former electoral district.[3] Hospitals had to be built according to a plan specified by the government. A typical cottage

* I have not been able to determine if settlement committees were ever appointed.

** Two more were constructed in the mid 1960s-Bell Island and Baie Verte. Surprisingly, Trepassey, at the southern tip of the Avalon Peninsula never rated a Cottage Hospital while Bell Island, only a short distance from St. John's, did.

hospital was a two-three-storey, usually a white painted wooden structure with a dispensary, delivery/operating room, out-patient clinic and accommodation for the staff. There were male and female wards for around ten patients, but for higher numbers in larger centres. In the early days the staff consisted of one physician, several nurses, a secretary treasurer, a janitor and several maids.[13]

A glaring deficiency in the Cottage Hospital plan in its earlier days, was the absence of microscopes and reagents to perform even the simplest tests. As late as 1941, I was told, there was only one microscope for all the hospitals. During the war the Director of Medical Laboratories and the Chief Radiologist at the General Hospital began to provide a combined course for training technicians in both radiography and simple laboratory procedures. Eventually all the Cottage Hospitals had two technicians and reasonable radiologic and laboratory equipment.

The accommodations provided for the staff were a source of endless complaints. The physician and his wife, if married, and nurses were all crowded into cramped quarters.[4] Obviously it would be difficult to attract and retain a physician, especially a married one, unless he was provided with a residence. Gradually these began to be built and furnished by raising funds locally and with support from the government. The physician would be charged a rent.[14, 15] Breakdowns in utilities were frequent. Running water might flow only intermittently and generators expired at the most inopportune times.[4] The Salaried Physicians Service included, besides Cottage Hospital physicians, District Medical Officers practising out of ambulatory Health Centres.*

Miller visited a Cottage Hospital every few years. In the days when he was DMS, he and Sir John Puddester would travel in style in a private railway coach, complete with a chef. A young physician travelling with them back to his Cottage Hospital remembers the contrast between the luxury of the private coach with its beautifully served breakfast on a white linen tablecloth with gleaming silver cutlery, and the squalor of the other coaches – the floors littered with discarded orange peels, crumpled newspaper and scraps of

•Over the years, the government took over the small hospitals at Buchans, Twillingate, Stephenville, Goose Bay, Grand Bank, St. Lawrence, Botwood and Gander. Miller recommended against acquiring the last two.[3] These new acquisitions ended in one strange imbalance – three hospitals at the tip of the Burin Peninsula!

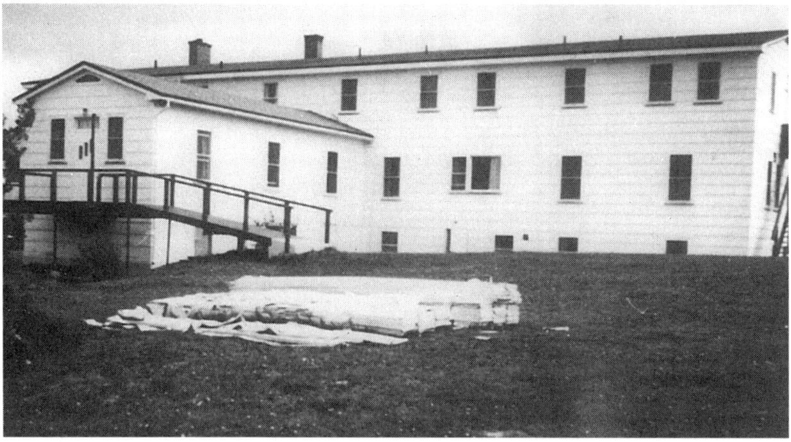

Old Perlican Cottage Hospital circa 1970
Courtesy Centre of Newfoundland Studies

food. Miller came to know every nook and cranny of each hospital. T.A. Hickman, a former Minister of Health recalls a request from a hospital for an expensive plan for renovations. Miller examined it. "They don't need this; by putting in a door here, and a wall there, they can get essentially what they want at half the cost."

The Cottage Hospital Scheme, was heavily dependent on physicians from the British Isles for its staff. For some reason it did not attract Mainlanders in any significant numbers . Newfoundland was the first port of call for many of the overseas physicians emigrating to Canada. Licensing requirements were easy. A physician could come to the island, work as a salaried physician for a few years, enough to fulfill national licensing requirements and then move on to another part of Canada. Consequently there was a high turnover rate. Every year Miller or another official would travel to London to sign up physicians for the plan. In the early postwar years there was no shortage of applicants, but as the years went by the number began to dwindle. L.E. Drake of the Medical Advisory Bureau of the British Medical Association, which the department used as its agency for recruiting, sounded this alarm bell: "As you know, I have over the past years, warned you of the steadily failing interest in posts [with the Newfoundland Department of Health] and we have now reached rock bottom."[16] One of the reasons he assigned for the declining interest in Newfoundland, was the salary scale which, while competitive with other parts of Canada, was not high enough.

Did Miller entice applicants to sign up for Cottage Hospitals under false pretences as has sometimes been alleged? A close physician friend of Miller's warned a young physician contemplating a Cottage Hospital posting, "If you do business with Miller, examine carefully any deal he offers; it almost invariably turns out to the department's advantage." But Miller could hardly be faulted for doing this. It would be a much graver charge if it can be shown that he deliberately mislead an applicant. There is nothing to show that he did. On the other hand, it is easy to understand that an applicant might fail to take in what he was being told or that he omitted to ask the right questions and then later came to believe that he had been misled. Obviously, Miller would not dwell on the drawbacks of a posting he was trying to sell. The evidence shows that Miller had the best interest of the applicant at heart. Dr. P. Warrick, after completing a locum in St. John's, went to see Miller about a Cottage Hospital posting. Miller advised against it pointing out that his children would soon be reaching an age when he would want them to have better educational opportunities than were available in the outports. What surprised several physicians was that after they left the Cottage Hospital system, Miller continued to take an interest in their careers and when he could, would send business their way.

In the long run, Miller believed that Newfoundland would have to depend on its own training programs to meet its needs.[17] In 1963, The student bursary program was extended to the second and third year premedical and predental students. Miller had great hopes that this would be the answer to the province's medical manpower shortage. The number of years the beneficiaries had to give to government service was equal to the years of support. The type of work the recipients of bursaries might be required to do varied in salary and interest, and this was a source of discontent and accusations of bad treatment. Some might be sent to Cottage Hospital positions but might find the accommodation unsatisfactory. Others might be required to do a series of locums to relieve Cottage Hospital doctors. Still others might spend all their time in St. John's in child welfare or maternal outpatient clinics. Only those who were sent to fill Cottage Hospital vacancies seemed to have been reasonably satisfied. One dental student wished to postpone returning to Newfoundland until after he completed post graduate studies.

Miller was firm at holding him to the terms of his bursary but, ever tactful and conciliatory, did it in a manner to soften his refusal and not to dash the students hopes. "I regret I cannot consent to your request to delay your return. Why not return for a couple of years and then take postgraduate work?"[18]

On the whole the bursary programs functioned reasonably satisfactory until medicare came, when there was a financial incentitive to break a contract, go into fee-for-service practice, where quick money was to be made, and pay back what was owing to the government. It was a great blow to Miller when several bursary recipients took this perfectly legal way out from their commitments.

It was the method of payment of salaried physicians which was to cause so much ill will and accusations of deals made secretly with individual doctors. In the early days salaries were computed on the basis of a percentage of the fees collected in a district plus a stipend from the government.[19] After 1956 salary scales for each post were introduced. The physician was allowed to keep fees collected from non-contractual services. The problem was that the department did not hesitate to abandon its own schedule of payments when it saw fit, as the following examples show.

The department proposed moving an MHO to another hospital as backup internist to a Senior Medical Officer who was also a surgeon. This involved a step down in rank for the MHO to the rank of a Senior Assistant Medical Officer and consequently a lower salary. To avoid this, the department saw that he was paid the salary of an MHO.[20] Sometimes a physician would be appointed at a lower salary scale than the minimum stipulated for the particular post because of "insufficient training or experience or workload."[21] A third example will suffice to show the disorder in salaries. A Cottage Hospital physician was told that if he stayed on, a special grade would be created for him. It was said that many a salaried physician left Miller's office with the impression that he was the favoured recipient of a special deal. No wonder Miller discouraged conclaves of physicians comparing salaries, but they did and some came to feel that they had been misled and hard done by. To give Miller his due, his aim appears to have been to factor in workload, special skills, and departmental needs in computing a salary. Unfortunately the end result was a chaotic system of payments that was so complicated that it was said only Miller knew the rationale behind each physician's salary. Not surprisingly he found himself accused of being Machiavellian by dividing and conquering. He referred to this common perception without comment: "You know we were always accused of doing separate deals with people – behind other peoples' backs – we never lived that down – true or not."[22]

It is to the department's credit that in the days before pensions it felt it had an obligation to find pensions for those who had spent a lifetime in the system, and for their widows.[23, 24] In the early days there was no provision for study leave and if a physician went on holidays he had to pay the travelling expenses of his replacement. The doctor was on call all the time. Only in the 1950s did the Department start the practice of staffing each hospital with at least two physicians.[25]

There was no defined chain of command at a Cottage Hospital; the doctor, head nurse and secretary-treasurer were supposed to work out a harmonious *modus vivendi* with the doctor in charge of admitting, treating and discharging patients. Sometimes Miller would be appealed to and asked to resolve a dispute. The decision to leave the chain of command undefined was deliberate.[3] To have designated a doctor as the one in command might have given umbrage to the secretary and head nurse.[3]

It was not only the terms of employment which caused vexation to salaried physicians. The people he was sent to serve could also give him trouble. A firm of management consultants observed that welfare payments had risen faster than earned incomes over the previous two decades and consequently it had become more profitable to stay on welfare.[26] The firm listed several deplorable consequences from this "welfare mentality". Patients would badger a social worker to give them taxi chits to visit a doctor in a larger center and then club together to go in one taxi on a shopping spree, the driver splitting the money from the taxi chits between himself and his passengers.[26] No wonder the Department was appalled at the amount of money it was dispensing on patient transportation. Physicians also reported patients being rude and threatening them for refusing to issue disability certificates.[27] Such behaviour could only widen the gulf between patients and their physicians and discourage doctors from staying.

Miller's interest in the salaried physicians did not end with their hiring. It is a measure of his farsightedness that he gave thought to their continuing medical education. As early as 1949 he wrote to Dr. Ian Rusted, who was doing postgraduate training in internal medicine, asking if he would assume responsibility for preparing postgraduate training programs for the salaried physicians. In his reply Rusted agreed, but suggested, *inter alia*, specialist consultant visits to the Cottage Hospitals.[28] Upon his return to Newfoundland in 1952 Rusted was employed by the Department of Health as a full-time, later part-time, consultant with a mandate to implement the programs he suggested. He enlisted the cooperation and support of the NMA and the Continuing Education Division of Dalhousie University.[28]

Both Miller and Rusted realized that it was useless to offer postgraduate training programs if physicians could not take time away from their duties. Miller tried to get around this obstacle by hiring one salaried physician to carry out rotating locums for physicians going on study leave. Later the department gradually began to place at least two physicians in each hospital.[25] In looking back at what was regarded as a program of extremely high calibre, Rusted admitted that "a great deal of the credit is due to Dr. Miller and his associates in the Department of Health for their strong support in these developments."[28]

As medicare approached, a major concern of the Department of Health was whether the salaried physicians might opt for fee for service, as would be their right. A management firm recommended that to avoid a mass exodus of salaried physicians, they should be offered a 35% increase in salary across the board.[29] The department settled for a 34% – 20% increase, depending on the position.[30] In addition, the department offered study leave and pensions. This package was attractive enough to persuade the salaried physicians as a bloc not to go 'fee for service'. An added incentive to accept the government's offer was the realization they would have to move out of their houses and furnish and equip their own offices.[31]

By the 1960s, criticisms of the Cottage Hospitals began to surface as the briefs to the Brain Commission demonstrated. The premiums had not kept pace with inflation. The department had realized this for a long time and would have liked to have seen a more realistic rate of increase over the years.[32] But a government as sensitive to public opinion as Smallwood's, hesitated. The rate of reimbursement for specialist care at the General Hospital for patients referred in from rural areas was ridiculously low. But the department was always chronically short of funds and without an infusion of federal funds could not afford to be more generous. Still, in spite of criticisms of the services they offered, there were no complaints about quality of care at the Cottage Hospitals.[33] The evidence seems to show that the Cottage Hospital Scheme, given the financial constraints under which it operated, did bring an acceptable level of care to rural Newfoundland. The scheme has been criticized for the lack of public involvement in its administration. This charge crops up both in the NMA brief to Lord Brain and the Report itself.[33,34]

By the mid-1960s the part of the Trans Canada Highway that traversed the island had been completed and work had started on branch roads to coastal communities. There were also redundancies due to the acquisition of other small hospitals. This should have been the time for a thorough revision of the network of Cottage Hospitals to determine which could be down-graded to " Nursing Stations" and which expanded into regional hospitals. The department was well aware that this should be done,[35] but again its hands were tied. Communities rise up in arms at any suggestion of closing or downgrading a hospital, and Smallwood was not going to court this sort of anger.*

Newfoundland is famed abroad for its Cottage Hospital Scheme. A dispassionate account of its operations cannot capture the flavour of its vivid lifelong impact on the lives of the many doctors and nurses who came to work in rural Newfoundland. The reminiscences of one Cottage Hospital physician succeed in picturing the joys and frustrations, the humour and the rewards of a Cottage Hospital doctor with Miller in the background minding his own business, leaving the doctor to work out things for himself, but available to advise or to settle contentious matters.

Noel Murphy, educated in England, was serving as a Squadron Leader in the RAF when he was surprised one day to receive a

* Two exceptions were the replacement of Stephenville Crossing and the IGA Hospital at Happy Valley by nearby hospitals at Stephenville and Goose Bay, acquired from the USA Armed Forces.

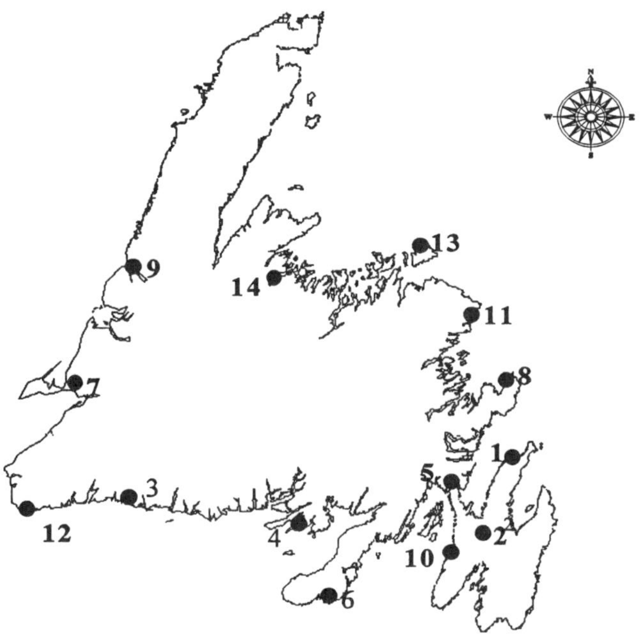

The Cottage Hospital Network in order of opening			
No.	Date	No.	Date
	1936		1940
1	Old Perlican	8	Bonavista
2	Markland	9	Norris Point
3	Burgeo		1942
4	Harbour Breton	10	Placentia
5	Come By Chance		1944
6	Burin	11	Brookfield
	1937		1952
7	Stephenville Crossing	12	Channel-Port-aux Basques
		13	Fogo Island
		14	Springdale

Courtesy D. Gordon, Department of Environment, Government of Newfoundland

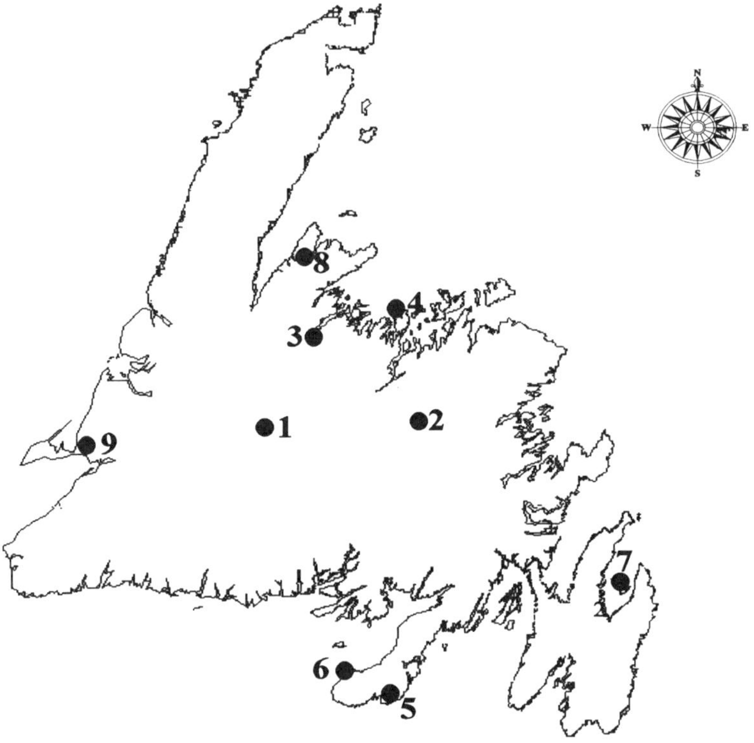

Cottage Hospitals Built or Aquired After 1952			
NO.	Place	No.	Place
1	Buchans	6	Grand Bank
2	Gander	7	Bell Island
3	Botwood	8	Baie Verte
4	Twillingate	9	Stephenville
5	St. Lawrence		

Courtesy D. Gordon, Department of Environment, Government of Newfoundland telegram from Miller, of whom he had never heard, asking if he would be willing to come home and take charge of the hospital at Norris Point, a scenic spot situated on a fjord on the west coast of the island and surrounded by high hills, snow-capped for much of the year. The war was drawing to its close and Murphy could see no reason for prolonging his service. He wired back "Yes" and his discharge was promptly arranged. Back in St. John's he was briefed by Miller on his duties and then taken over to be introduced to Sir John Puddester. While they were waiting outside Puddester's office, someone said to Murphy, " That is a man you will never see 'eye to eye' with." This got Murphy really worried. When Miller and Murphy went into the office, Puddester had his head down and continued writing for a minute or so. He then lifted up his head and Murphy grasped the point of the warning he had just received. Puddester was cross-eyed. Miller who had overheard the remark looked at the amused Murphy, but never cracked a smile. After the introduction, Murphy and his wife were dispatched to St. Clare's Hospital to learn the intricacies of operating an X-Ray machine and developing films; for in those days wives were supposed to assist their husbands in their work (without pay of course!). As a solo physician, Murphy found himself doing everything from urinalysis to emergency operations. He had no holiday for five years because there was no one to relieve him. Every two or three years Miller would come on a visit, preceeded by a telegram announcing the date and time of arrival, usually by boat.

Once Murphy came with him on a plane which developed engine trouble. Miller didn't show the slightest sign of fear. The first item on Miller's agenda for the hospital visit was to sound out the wife about her feelings towards her husband's job. If she was discontented, as he used to say, it would be a waste of time talking to the husband. Fortunately, Murphy's wife always gave the right responses. Miller then would tour the hospital. This was no cursory inspection, but more like a captain inspecting his ship. His practised eye took in everything. Time would then be set aside to talk to the head nurse to see how she was getting on with the doctor and to meet with the chairman of the local health committee. Finally, Miller looked through the log book, which recorded every item of medical and surgical service on a daily basis, to get an idea of the doctor's work load.

While Miller's visits, were always looked forward to, the same could not be said of the visits of the multitude of carping bureaucrats who came to check on the doctor's activities and who were usually totally ignorant of local conditions. Why did he not keep medications under lock and key? Why didn't he test the water etc.? The answers were simple. The people were honest and theft was unheard of. What would be the point of testing the water, because there was nothing Murphy could do about it if it was bad.

The territory Murphy was responsible for was large, extending up and down the coast for more than one hundred kilometres . When things were quiet at the hospital, he would go on visits to the outlying communities, travelling in summer by cabin cruiser and in winter by dogsled. It is difficult to realize how unsophisticated the people were in those days. Many, having used only an outhouse, had never seen a toilet. Murphy remembers sending a patient into the hospital lavatory to produce a sample of urine. On coming out the patient said, "Sir, I've never seen a spring coming out of the floor before."

Chronic shortage of funds was an ever present handicap. The automatic response to any request out of the ordinary was 'no'. Murphy asked for a cystoscope, reasoning that this would be a saving since patients requiring cystoscopy had to be to sent to St. John's. He got the stock answer from Miller that if he gave him one he would have to do the same for other Cottage Hospital physicians. To which Murphy replied, "What if I raise half the cost?" Quickly the answer came back, " I don't have any choice, do I? I have to go along with it." This is an example of what many have told me, that if a physician was enthusiastic about a scheme and could convince Miller of its worth and showed some initiative in its implementation, he could count on Miller's support – especially if he could raise part of the required funds! On another occasion Murphy asked for screens for his house, only to get the usual refusal. Anyone knowing a Newfoundland summer and its hords of biting insects, can sympathize with Murphy when he replied that in that case he would have to leave. This was enough for Miller. A few weeks later a letter arrived from the Department of Public Works saying the screens would be supplied.

But like so many Cottage Hospital physicians who enjoyed their work and its style of life, the time came when Murphy had to leave because his children had reached an age requiring educational opportunities that were not available at Norris Point.

After all these years, Murphy looks back to Miller with respect and affection for his unfailing support. It was the famous smile which stands out. "It was a fleeting smile that came and went, smile again and then go blank, you never knew if he was enjoying it or not or what it was, otherwise he always wore a solemn look. He was honest, more honest then he needed to be, he was very dedicated and anxious to help as much as possible, but the dollar always stood in the way of giving people what they wanted. He also left you alone to do your job but was available if needed."

One day Murphy was surprised to receive a telegram, out of the blue, from Miller saying a snowmobile was on its way. He hadn't asked for one. This was entirely Miller's doing. He had been able to get it through the NHGP. For Murphy this was typical of Miller's thoughtfulness. He knew Murphy had to cover long distances and that in winter a snowmobile would be a great improvement over a dogsled.

Murphy praises Miller for his skill in settling disputes. He once had to call on Miller to resolve a conflict with the Head Nurse, who was encroaching into his area of responsibility. On this occasion action was required rather than diplomacy, and a transfer of the nurse was promptly arranged.

Murphy's resignation from the Cottage Hospital system did not end his friendship with Miller. They kept in touch with each other over the years and Miller would drop in to see him when he was in Corner Brook.

Sufficient time has elapsed for those who were served by the Cottage Hospital Scheme to make their own assessment of its worth. But how should the performance of the one who presided over it for so many years be rated? Many have testified to his honest, quiet, competent day-by-day administration of a system, always plagued by a shortage of funding and staff. He certainly campaigned to redress these deficiencies. On the other hand he never pushed for a radical restructuring of the whole system.

Chapter 15 – Notes

1. Newfoundland Royal Commission 1933 HM Stationary Office Kingsway, London WC2.

2. Lewis, J.E.C. *Nursing Service, Preventive and Curative.* Canadian Hospital 39 (2):55-56 1962.

3. NRC Miller, L.A. *History of Cottage Hospitals* (An address to the Medical History Society October 9, 1980) Unpublished .

4. Miller, L.A. *The Cottage Hospital Plan in Newfoundland.* Newfoundland Medical Association Newsletter 16 (4): 23-27 1974.

5. McConaghey, R.M.S. *The Evolution of the Cottage Hospital.* Medical History 11:128-140, 1967.

6. Rompkey, Ronald. *Grenfell of Labrador. A Biography.* University of Toronto Press. Toronto 1991. P.106.

7. Rompkey R. ibid P. 168-169.

8. PANL Newfoundland Royal Commission of Health and Public Charities. First Interim Report. St. John's. Kings Printer. June 1930.

9. PANL Cottage Hospital Scheme GN 38 S6-1-1 (Undated). ?1934.

10. ANLMA LAM to ARM 1962-12-21.

11. CNS JCCC. No date No Author.

12. ANLMA LAM to NMA Ex Comm. 1953 -02-5 .

13. McCarthy M. *Day to Day Experiences of a Nurse in Charge.* Canadian Hospital 39 (2): 57, 86 1962.

14. CNS JRSC JMcG Memo 1958-08-28.

15. CNS JRSC JMcG Memo 1959-03-03.

16. CNS JRSC LED to JMcG1967-05-02.

17. CNS JCCC LAM to J McG 1967-02-10.

18. PANL Box 9361 Health LAM to RQ 1967-02-08.

19. CNS JRSC J McG Memo 1961-10-23.

20. CNS JRSC J McG Memo 1964-05-12.

21. CNS Health 5-'69 TAH Memo 1969-02-04.

22. NRC Miller, L.A. Memoir unpublished.

23. CNS JRSC JMcG Memo 1961-10-23.

24. CNS JRSC J McG Memo 1962-5-02.

25. Miller L.A. *Cottage Hospital System* . Canadian Hospital 39 (2): 48-49 1962.

26. CNS JCCC Kates, Peat, Marwick, Report on Cottage Hospitals 1968.

27. CNS JRSC JR to WPC 1971 -3-1.

28. Rusted, I. *Recollections of Continuing Medical Education in Newfoundland.* Newfoundland Medical Association Newsletter 18 (1): 5-9 1976.

29. CNS JCCC Kates, Peat, Marwick, RAD to JCC 1968-04-01.

30. CNS JRSC TAH Memo 1968-12-6

31. ANLMA NMA Reps. and J. McG and LAM 1967-08-28.

32. CNS JRSC JRC to JRS 1952-08-29.

33. *NMA Recommendations to Royal Commission on Health.* Newfoundland Medical Association Newsletter 7 (3):9 1965.

34. Royal Commission on Health, Right Honourable Lord Brain 1966 Vol. 1 p. 22.

35. PANL PRC 19 35- 1-6- 1 WPC to LAM Re. Inclusions in Brief of the Department of Health to Royal Commission on Health. 1965 -03-27.

CHAPTER 16

Private Hospitals

During Miller's day, there were several non-government owned acute care hospitals in the province, two in St. John's: St. Clare's Hospital, operated by the Sisters of Mercy and The Grace General Hospital owned by the Salvation Army, and one each in Grand Falls and Corner Brook.

In the first two decades after Confederation the population of the city of St. John's tripled and with it a sizeable middle-class grew which looked to the two private hospitals for in-patient care. The Grace and St. Clare's hospitals both expanded to supply their needs. Some of the returning specialists, dissatisfied with conditions at the General Hospital, gravitated to the Grace. By so doing they were cut off from treating referrals from the Cottage Hospitals which had to be sent to the General. Even though the fees were low this annoyed the specialists at the Grace and St. Clare's and they lobbied to have the policy changed. This was another source of friction with the Department of Health which adamantly restated its commitment to "the policies that the General be the main referral centre [from the Cottage Hospitals]."[1] Of course medicare put an end to restrictions on referrals from the Cottage Hospitals, but the General was able to maintain its lead as the chief referral centre for the province by its transformation into the university hospital, albeit still under its old name, in a brand new building on the university campus. During his last years in office, Miller was occupied in working on this change and the terms of affiliation with the medical school; he must surely deserve some of the credit for its satisfactory outcome.

The government was not involved in the operations of the two private hospitals in St. John's until 1958 when federal/provincial hospital insurance was enacted. The government then began to exercise increasing control over their operations as they became more dependent on government funding. This led to arguments on a number of occasions between the Department of Health and the private hospitals. One cause of friction was a hospital's unwillingness to accept government-imposed conditions on shared cost items. A dispute arose between the Administrator of the Grace Hospital and the Department over the terms of appointment of a part-time Medical Director. The Administrator insisted that the terms of appointment were to be determined only by the hospital's Board of Management and categorically rejected the terms stipulated by the Department.[2] The Administrator then wrote over the head of Miller to McGrath and received this reply: "I cannot subscribe to the theory that this Department will have no control over the type of services rendered where appointments are made for which we supply funds."[3]

Another cause of concern to government, was that as hospital staffs became unionized, each hospital made its own deal with unions contrary to government policy, which was to have the same salaries for posts of similar grade and seniority across the province.[4, 5]

Perhaps the most frequent cause of hard feelings, after 1958, was the difficulty hospital boards found in keeping disbursements within the funds allocated by the government. Hospitals were tempted to disregard budgetary controls, running up debts and then looking to the government to bail them out.[6] On one occasion the Board of Management of the Western Memorial Hospital, Corner Brook, proposed exceeding its budget in spite of departmental warnings.[7] Miller, who was *ex officio* a member of the board, was present at the meeting when this decision was made. He was never one to be caught in the position of being a lone stalwart facing an angry shouting crowd. Confrontation had to be avoided at all costs. To extricate himself from a potentially acrimonious situation, he advised the Board to defer any action until he had returned to St. John's and had had an opportunity to discuss the matter with the Minister.[8] The Board agreed. The Minister then wrote to the hospital administrator pointing out the obvious folly of Board's going into debt.[9] The Board backed down.

Since the two private hospitals in St. John's were owned by two different religious groups, this led to a certain amount of rivalry. The government could not bestow a favour on one without the other knocking on its door for the same benefit. This consideration was always uppermost in Miller's mind in responding to a request from one or the other. It was particularly difficult to satisfy both the Grace and St. Clare's in the last years of the Smallwood era when, under pressure from its bankers, the government had agreed to a strict borrowing policy.[10] This was just the time when one of the private hospitals (hospital A) chose to expand and requested government assistance, arguing that the other private hospital (hospital B) had received generous support for its expansion some years earlier. What then happened is a tribute to Smallwood's ability to extricate himself from an embarrassing mess of his own making.

Smallwood had publicly committed the government to help the expansion of hospital A with a large grant. Shortly afterwards the Minister of Finance told the Premier that there were no funds to meet the pledge. Subsequently, the budget for that year contained no reference to the expansion grant. Time went by. The Minister of Health and Miller were both uneasy that the hospital had not been told the bad news. The impatient Minister kept reminding Smallwood that he should break the news to the executive director of the hospital as soon as possible. Smallwood refused and ordered the Minister to undertake this unenviable task himself. The minister called the executive director and broke the bad news. It was a horrible experience. In his words, "anger, prejudice, accusations of going back on one's word etc." Still, the job had been done. The bullet had been bitten. That weekend the Minister was surprised to be called at his home by the Premier, a most unusual event. A bizarre conversation then took place, more or less along the following lines:

Premier: Minister, there has been a rumour that [hospital A] is not able to proceed with its building program this year. I don't know how the rumour got out.

Minister of Health: Well, you know how it got out. We decided at a Cabinet Meeting that we did not have the funds for the hospital's expansion. You told me to tell the executive director and I did so. It is not a rumour.

At this point in the story the Minister observed, "I began to notice that he was talking as if I were not there and I wondered if it was for the benefit of somebody in the room."

Min.: Mr. Premier, is there someone in the room with you?

Premier: Yes, X and dear old Y who has crawled out of a sick bed. They had heard the rumour and came to see me to be assured that it was false. I told them it was not true.

Min.: But it is true. The Cabinet agreed there is no money for the extension, not even the token dollar which would have allowed the government to keep it on their books.

Premier: I know what you're saying Minister; you are so right. I knew you would come up with the answer. We have no money to give the hospital this year, but I take your advice. They can borrow the dollars that are necessary to start the extension this year and the government will guarantee the loan.

Min.: No, Mr. Premier, that's not what I am saying. That is still a charge against the government.

Premier.: You are so right again, Minister. They can borrow the money as you say and the government will guarantee the loan. I will tell these two gentlemen. They will be forever grateful to you.

Then the Premier hung up.

The next day the Minister of Health recounted this strange conversation to Miller who asked him what he planned to do. He replied, "Nothing. I suppose if I were the Minister of Finance, I would resign."

As far back as 1945 Miller had argued, in a memorandum to Puddester, that government should have its own hospital expansion program policy.[11] To leave it up to individual hospitals to decide when to expand and then to come for funding to the government was to put the government always on the defensive. Unfortunately, the Smallwood government never developed a coherent rational hospital construction and renovation program. Everything was left to political whim. But Miller, in spite of his wise advice to Puddester, does not appear to have taken steps himself to initiate a master-plan for hospital construction. Like Smallwood, he put himself in the position of responding to a request for expansion for a new hospital rather than being its proposer. At Carbonear the initiative for a 20-bed hospital came entirely from the community.[12] Miller was supportive of the idea and guided the local committee through the planning stage, suggesting they begin simply with out-patient and diagnostic services before proceeding to construct a 20-bed hospital. This figure was chosen because at that time The Canadian Red Cross was equipping, furnishing and operating hospitals of this size in remote areas of Canada. The Red Cross approved the plans for the hospital and took over its operations.

Miller played a passive but guiding role in the fund-raising campaign for the Carbonear Hospital and in its construction. He was supportive and helpful in his advice. He knew the Red Cross was equipping, furnishing and operating 20-bed community hospitals in remote regions, yet there is nothing to show that he took any steps to spur other communities to imitate Carbonear or to tap this source himself. He certainly argued for a hospital building master-plan in the Department's brief to Lord Brain,[13] but he obviously believed that the initiative should come from the government, and not from him.

In the last year of the Smallwood government some order and method was put into the renovation of old hospitals and the building of new ones by the institution of a joint planning committee for each new project.[14] The Minister of Health nominated the members of the committee in consultation with the Minister of Public Works and included representatives of the relevant Hospital Board. The committee was charged with the selection of an architect and supervision of construction of the building. Public tenders were advertised, the award going to the lowest bidder unless there were good reasons to the contrary.

Chapter 16 – Notes

1. CNS JCCC LAM to JCC 1968-02-09.

2. CNS JRSC ADM to LAM 1966-03-29.

3. CNS JRSC J McG to ADM 1966-05-05.

4. CNS JRSC Executive Council Memo 1964-02-22.

5. CNS JRSC JMcG to JRS 1964-01-13.

6. CNS JCCC LM to JCC 1967-10-26.

7. CNS RJB to CAS 1969-12-15.

8. CNS LAM to ER 1969-12-23.

9. CNS ER to LM 1970-01-07.

10. CNS EMRC DP to JRS 1969-05-22.

11. PANL GN38 S6-5-2 LAM to JCP 1945-10-4.

12. Rowe A.T. *Carbonear Blueprint for the Future* Newfoundland Medical Association Newsletter 6(2): 12-14 1964.

13. PANL PRC 19 Health Box 35161 Brief of Department of Health to Royal Commission on Health. 1965-08-19.

14. CNS Department of Health Memo 27-'70.

CHAPTER 17

The Newfoundland Medical Association

Liaison Committee and the Annual General Meeting.

Prior to the Cottage Hospital system there was little occasion for conflict between the NMA and the government of the day. But as the number of physicians paid wholly or in part by government increased and the NMA became their advocate, disputes between the Association and the Department of Health started to arise. Following Confederation, as the government began to assume increasing responsibility for the health care of the entire province, it was obliged to give more time and attention to its relations with the NMA.

Miller appreciated the importance of getting the support or at least the tacit acquiescence of the NMA for new government policies. He never forgot that he was a physician and he saw himself as a bridge between government and doctors. It is a tribute to his diplomatic skills that he was able to establish a satisfactory working relationship with the NMA which, although sometimes strained, continued amicably up to his retirement. While not all the physicians would have concurred with the following somewhat fulsome encomium which appeared in the official organ of the association, it probably expressed the considered opinion of the majority, at least of Miller: "One cannot help being impressed by doctors McGrath and Miller, those two father figures, these elder statesmen, who have been directing the Health Department for so many years. Both are wise, earnest men and their opinions, which do not court popularity, must be given full consideration."[1]

There were two avenues through which Miller maintained communication with the Association. The first was through meetings with the Liaison Committee of the NMA, and the second was attendance at the AGM of the Association.

Miller seems to have been the first to take the initiative by urging the NMA to form a liaison committee to discuss matters of interest between NMA and the Minister and Deputy Minister of Health acting on behalf of the government.[2] It appears that Miller expected the NMA to call the meetings and prepare the agenda. Meetings were arranged on an ad hoc basis whenever the NMA had concerns, and long periods might elapse without any meeting. Miller would then prod the Association into calling one.[3] The place of meetings was sometimes a cause of disagreement. If the issues to be discussed were going to be contentious, neither party wished to put itself at the psychological disadvantage of meeting on the other party's turf.[4, 5] They would then agree to meet on neutral ground.

It took some years to establish an acceptable format for these meetings. In the early years, the Department tended to use them as a forum for announcing government policy, with no room for discussion or negotiation. Dr. James McGrath, the long-time Minister of Health and a somewhat blustery, overbearing man on occasions, was particularly prone to act in this way and once the NMA delegates became so incensed that they called for an immediate adjournment. Dr. W.D. Parsons, an NMA representative at these meetings recalls their order. In the days when Dr. J. McGrath was minister of health, the leader of the NMA delegation would address McGrath saying they wished to have an update report on a particular project. McGrath would reply with, "Yes, it is going well. Len, are we having any problems with such and such?" Miller would then take over and provide the detailed background information. As a consummate politician Miller always let the suggestions come from McGrath. The same NMA representative had the impression that McGrath and Miller had discussed the agenda before the meeting and had settled how each topic was to be handled. Relations were always close between the two men and McGrath never felt any need to put Miller down. Other

Ministers were not so secure in themselves. One Minister insisted on carrying the ball entirely himself, practically excluding Miller, and another took care to run the meetings but referred to Miller from time to time. Miller, with his accustomed aplomb, adapted his ways to those of whoever was the incumbent Minister and was always careful to stay in the background until called upon by him. The NMA seems to have found Miller most obliging in providing it with information upon request.[6] The Department of Health could test the waters at these meetings which were the ideal venue for passing on sensitive information and probing the reaction of the profession to proposed new policies . But for all parties to feel free to say what they wanted, it was essential that the proceedings be kept confidential. This became a bone of contention, the NMA arguing that points were brought up repeatedly and then nothing was done about them. For a time anyway, it was agreed to take minutes of the proceedings, but to keep them under lock and key.[7] Still, at the liaison meetings Miller was able to generate an atmosphere of trust and freedom: "It is very gratifying to all concerned that close cooperation with Dr. Miller and his Assistants has enabled the Association to feel free to discuss outstanding matters and arrive at conclusions satisfactory to all." [7]

In 1960 the NMA wrote to Miller proposing replacing the Liaison Committee with bimonthly meetings between the Minister, Deputy Minister and Executive Committee of the NMA, the Executive Committee to be considered as an advisory health committee to the Minister as required by the Children's Health Plan.[8] The Minister agreed to this suggestion, and for the remainder of Miller's career the Executive Committee of the NMA also fulfilled a liaison role with the Department.[9]

To Miller, the NMA was more than just the official representative of the physicians, to be cajoled into acquiesence by government initiatives. It was a valuable resource to be consulted on social and health issues. For example, how should addicts be handled who visited multiple physicians to obtain prescriptions for narcotics?[10] At the Minister of Health's request, the NMA advised on what should be done with the Fort Pepperell Hospital when the Americans turned over the base to Canadian authorities. Its recommendations were approved by McGrath and Miller, but not by Smallwood (See Chapter 8).

If the Department of Health was to discharge its duties efficiently it had to know what the doctors were thinking and what were their concerns. For Miller there was no better way of becoming informed on these points than by attending the AGM of the NMA, which he did punctiliously up to his death long after his retirement. For many years he would be the luncheon speaker on the last day of the business part of the meeting. His speech would take the form of a " state of the union" address reviewing the achievements of the Department during the past year and unveiling plans for the year to come. They were eagerly awaited by the physicians.

The officers of the Association came and went while Miller remained at the helm for years. This placed them at a disadvantage. None could match him in administrative skills or experience. At the business meetings he did not participate much in the debates, but would intervene to point out flaws or inconsistencies in a report that would have escaped the less experienced eyes of the officers of the Association.[11]

The majority of physicians recognized that his innate wisdom and long years of experience gave him the authority to warn the Association when it might be embarking on an unwise course of action. On one occasion a misguided resolution was amended along the lines he suggested.[12] But at times he could be scathing in his comments. He once recommended that a report be rejected because it represented only one man's opinion and was biased.[13] A member protested, accusing the Deputy Minister of committing the same fault himself on occasions. Miller shot back, "Did the member imply that he had no right to express an opinion, and was he not free to say what he wanted unless silenced?"

The Association recognized that while Miller did not always do what it wanted, he was able to provide valid arguments for not doing so and that he had their best interests at heart. Over the years the NMA and the Department of Health enjoyed good relations, to the envy of other provinces, but they were not always harmonious. There was an undercurrent of discontent with certain policies of the Department and from time to time disputes erupted, but there was never a complete breach of relations although on several occasions they became distinctly chilly.

Cottage Hospital Referrals

A constant source of complaint was the amount of payments from government to physicians for patients referred to the General Hospital from the Cottage Hospitals. By 1963 this was 30% of the 1962 NMA schedule of fees.[14] This seemed to be a ridiculously low scale of payment to the Executive of the NMA and it passed a resolution requesting that it be increased to 90% of the NMA's schedule.[14] Miller replied with a refusal but left the door open for further negotiations.[15] In a later letter, with his usual careful choice of words, Miller had this to say: "While I can by no means assure you that it would be possible to grant an increase in fees–at the present time there might be some chance if you could go part way this year. The figure I had in mind is 60% of the fee schedule."[16] They eventually settled for this amount.[17]

Another complaint from the NMA was the refusal of the government to pay speciality fees for patients referred to the General Hospital who had not paid their annual premiums. The department's justification for this policy was that to pay for such cases would be to treat non subscribers as subscribers which would be an incentive for people not to pay their premiums.[18] This forced specialists, for humanitarian reasons, to treat such cases free of charge. Miller acknowledged that "we have never been able to find a proper solution to this problem". However, as he pointed out, the Department did not have the funds to pay for referral services on non-subscribers and advised stalling until medicare would take care of the problem.[19, 20]

The Oath

A major clash between the NMA and the Department of Health while Miller was Deputy Minister, occured over the Oath of Office, enacted in 1958.[21] The Act required all full-time employees of the government to take two oaths, one of allegiance and the other of secrecy. The salaried physicians came within the terms of the Act. The NMA raised objections to both oaths (many of the doctors were Irish), but it was the Oath of Secrecy which was the major bone of contention. The Association contended that it was incompatible with patent-physician confidentiality, clashed with the Hippocratic Oath and inhibited freedom of speech of Cottage Hospital physicians.[22]

At the 1960 AGM of the Association a resolution was passed requesting withdrawal of the Oath*, and failing this, petitioning the Legislative Assembly to change the Act to state that salaried physicians were not civil servants and exempt from the provisions of the Act.[22] In the discussion, Miller said he would abstain from voting on the resolution, stating that the Minister had been trying for years to obtain pensions for the Cottage Hospital doctors and that this would be possible only if they were incorporated into the civil service and that declaring them not to be civil servants would frustrate his efforts on their behalf. Nevertheless the NMA insisted in pursuing its efforts to implement the resolution and denied the argument of the Department of Health that pensionability depended upon being a civil servant.[23] The two parties received contradictory legal advice. The lawyers for the NMA and the CMA assured them that Cottage Hospital physicians were not civil servants while the Attorney General's department told the Minister of Health that they were.[24]

The Association's legal advisors suggested that the only way to clarify the status of Cottage Hospital doctors would be through a test case in the courts.[24] This course was favoured by the Executive Committee, but it soon found to its disappointment there was apathy among the salaried physicians about the Oath and reluctance to take any action. Perhaps they were more concerned with obtaining pensions than theoretical discussions about the incompatibility between an Oath of Secrecy and the Hippocratic Oath. The dispute dragged on for years. Lord Brain recommended that the Oath be rescinded.[25] It seems then to have been quietly dropped. Writing about the dispute years later, Miller relates that he was pushing for the Cottage Hospital doctors having to take the Oath so that they would be regarded as full-fledged civil servants and therefore pensionable.[26] He mentions his surprise at his efforts being so misunderstood.

"The Burin Situation"

Another time in the Miller era that relations between the NMA and the Department became strained, took place in the autumn of 1963. It raised questions which are as relevant today as then. Both

* It is not clear what the NMA was approving. The "whereas" parts and the resolution mention only the "Oath of Secrecy" while the " Be it Resolved" section refers to "the Oath." Presumably the NMA was calling for the rescinding of the dual Oath or exclusion of the salaried physicians from its terms. This is not made clear throughout the interminable debate.

parties gave press releases recounting their version of the events.[28] The facts of the case in "The Burin Situation," as it came to be referred to by the NMA, appear to be these.[29, 30]

Two pregnant women were admitted to the Burin Cottage Hospital with uterine bleeding. The admitting physician diagnosed each as an inevitable abortion and ordered ergotamine. The head nurse countermanded the orders (after one dose had been given) without informing the physician. When the latter found out what the nurse had done, he called Dr. W. Collingwood, Consultant, Treatment Services in the Department of Health, and who happened to be in the vicinity (Miller and McGrath were away). Collingwood came over two days later and gave his opinion that he would not have given ergotamine.[29, 30, 31] The treating physician and his colleague, according to their testimony, then asked Collingwood if this was an order "not to give ergotamine" and were told "it was"[30] (presumably this was a directive not to use ergotamine in the future in cases similar to these two patients). They replied that they would not take this order from Collingwood and furthermore demanded an apology from the offending nurse and assurances that she would not countermand orders again.[30] She refused. A few days later Collingwood wrote to the first of the two physicians " to confirm my verbal instructions" about the management of the cases and added that "this opinion has been confirmed by the obstetricians practicing in the city."[32] Collingwood then briefed Miller, who had returned to the province, on the facts of the affair.[30] Subsequently the two physicians contacted Collingwood and asked what the Department now proposed doing and were told, so they said, "nothing but the order not to give ergotamine still stood."[30] The two then tended their resignations, which were accepted.[27, 29, 30] A few days later, they went on the air and gave their version of the story, but focused only on the countermanding of their orders by the nurse. [33]

The fat was now in the fire. Because of widespread public debate over the dispute, the NMA had no choice but to become involved, even though the two physicians were not members of the Association.* The physicians were contacted and interviewed by the Executive Committee. Subsequently, the Minister of Health was asked to give permission for access to the records of the two

* Compulsory membership in the NMA was not mandatory for all practising physicians at that time.

patients.[30] A motion was also passed by the Executive Committee authorizing the secretary to contact Collingwood to ask him to discuss "this disturbing incident" with the Executive Committee.[30] There is no record of whether he availed himself of the invitation and no reply was received for the request to see the patients' records. The Association also sought the opinion of a group of gynecologists[34] and was assured that the two physicians had acted "in full accord with accepted practice."[29]

Meanwhile, the Minister of Health, in a press release, gave the Department's side of the story. He conceded that "under no circumstances is a nurse justified in omitting to advise a doctor when she has cancelled or refused to carry out an order."[27] He then went on to add that the policy of the Department of Health regarding the management of uterine bleeding in pregnancy had "always been that there should be no interference whatsoever with a pregnancy in whatever stage, unless there is an absolute necessity – in the presence of active danger to the patient." The Minister then said that "from the doctor's [sic] own notes. . . I'm of the opinion that an urgent necessity for the giving of ergotamine did not exist, but it is not suggested that the doctor's [sic] action was indefensible, in fact no action was taken or contemplated against the doctor [sic] . . . the doctors [sic] were advised of the Department's policy in such matters and instructions were given to follow a more conservative line of treatment in future cases . . . the doctors' [sic] reaction was to send in their resignations coupled with a clear indication that they refused to accept the principal that the Department had any right to give them any instructions whatever regarding medical treatment. The Minister is responsible for the care of patients in government hospitals . . . and must exercise the right to indicate his disapproval of certain lines of treatment."[27]

At this point the Association thought it should hear the offending nurse's version of events.

The secretary (following informal discussions with two members of the Executive Committee) called her and asked if she would be willing to give her side of the case.[35] She agreed, but a few hours later withdrew her consent. Shortly afterwards, Miller telephoned and asked the Association's secretary if it was true that he had asked the nurse to make a statement to the Executive Committee.

The secretary replied that it was true, and then Miller asked him if he could see anything improper in this behavior. He replied 'no,' and Miller made no further comment.[35] A few days later a furious letter arrived from the Minister, expressing outrage at the NMA asking the nurse to appear before the Executive Committee for interrogation.[36] He went on to add, "I do not consider that the Committee had any status in this matter or any right to interrogate this Department with its employees."

The reader will observe that the Minister's and the two physicians' accounts of events, don't quite tally. The Ministerial press release leaves the impression that the physicians' management of the cases had only been censured and that they had been cautioned to be more conservative in future.[27] Collingwood's letter is less clear,[32] but the two physicians were quite adamant that Collingwood had ordered them not to give ergotamine.[30] It was the claim, in the press release, that the Minister had a measure of control over the way a government-employed physician should practise, which troubled the NMA. Legal advice was sought. The opinion was given that because Cottage Hospital physicians were practising their profession under contract with the government, then the Department was entitled to exercise "a measure of general control and supervision."[37] A second legal opinion added that while the Minister could not dictate to a physician how to treat a particular case, the laws of the land did circumscribe modes of practice in particular situations such as compulsory immunization.[38]

These opinions are not too enlightening. It would have been more helpful if the lawyers had categorized medical acts into those which come under the heading of malpractice and those where there is diversity of medical opinion on management. No one would contest the right, indeed obligation of the department, to step in when one of its physicians is guilty of what could be construed as negligent or culpable mismanagement. In the case of the second category, the right of the department to dictate a particular line of treatment in preference to another, as it was accused by the two physicians of doing; this is a dubious proposition in a multi-confessional system such as the Cottage Hospital Scheme. Ultimately it is up to the licensing authorities and the courts to rule on what is or is not acceptable practice. But the department in its press release tacitly admitted that the actions of the two physicians fell into the second category, with the department and the two physicians advocating different lines of treatment and each able to cite reputable authorities to support its case. Left unsaid was the very obvious awareness by all that this was a case where therapeutic judgement could be influenced by religious convictions and this was the reason why passions were being aroused.

As time passed and tempers cooled the NMA began to become concerned about "alienation" [39] from the Department and quietly let the affair drop.

What is one to make of this fracas? It blew up in the first place because of Collingwood's blunders. Whether as a result of this incident or not, Miller, according to an official in the Department, had little confidence in Collingwood as an administrator. He could not dismiss him, but tended to sidetrack him. When it comes to assigning blame, neither the NMA nor the Department can be exonerated. Certainly the decision to invite the offending nurse to appear before the Executive Committee of the NMA, should have been a decision of the full committee and not one of several members acting on their own, and should have been subject to the permission of the Minister. But the conduct of the Department of Health is also blameworthy. It was wrong for the Minister to claim that the dispute was an internal matter and of no concern to others. Once it had become a matter of public debate and concern, the NMA had no choice but to become involved. If the department wished to appear even-handed, it was not enough just to express disapproval of the nurse's countermanding an order and failing to notify the physician; like the two doctors she should have been reprimanded and cautioned not to do it again. Again, in his press release, the Minister said that "the Department's policy has always been that there should be no interference in a pregnancy unless . . . in the presence of active danger to the patient."[27] He was being less than candid since no such policy had ever been enunciated, either verbally or in writing[31] – and wisely so. To have imposed such a ruling on the salaried physicians would have raised an outcry, apart from the difficulty of applying such an unworkable dictum, as the Minister had enunciated in his press release, to a particular clinical situation.

Left unsettled was the question whether the Department was only reprimanding the two physicians and advising them to be more conservative in the future - something within its rights, or whether it was giving orders how they were to act in similar situations in the future. The only way to have resolved the ambiguity would have been for the NMA to have put the question before the department, what action it would take against the two physicians if, after the reprimand and warning, they had continued to treat future cases of antepartum bleeding the same way they had done in the past. If the answer had been 'dismissal', this would have confirmed the Association's worst fears.

How does Miller come out of this affair? Early on when asked, he refused to comment.[33] He may have been inhibited in expressing his real thoughts because of his relationship with McGrath who was a practising Roman Catholic. He wisely stayed quietly in the background throughout the quarrel, although later he was quoted as having spoken publicly to the effect that the nurse was "justified in her action."[33, 39] There is no way now of knowing what interpretation to put upon this statement or even if he did ever make it. But certainly in light of the ministerial press release which criticized the nurse for cancelling an order and not notifying the physician, it would be inconceivable that he was approving of this conduct. The reason why the nurse was not disciplined, was because of the religious overtones to the dispute.* Presumably, and perhaps understandably, the Department did not want to stir up a hornet's nest and thought it wiser to take no action against her.

Looking back years later, with passions subsided, one is left with the impression that if the two parties to the dispute, instead of issuing missives and countermissives and listening to hearsay, had sat down together in the same room, they might have been able to sort out exactly what they were arguing about.

* A strange omission in this debate is the absence of any reference to the outcome in the two cases of antepartum bleeding.

Chapter17 – Notes

1. Newfoundland Medical Association Newsletter 9 (3)1967.

2. ANLMA LAM to CHP Sec NMA 1951 -09-22.

3. ANLMA Ex Comm NMA 1952-10-16.

4. ANLMA Ex Comm NMA 1957-12-20.

5. ANLMA Ex Comm NMA 1960-01-20.

6. ANLMA LAM to DB 1961-01-25.

7. ANLMA Sec. Report NMA 1960-06-02,3,4.

8. ANLMA CUH to LAM 1960-09-28.

9. ANLMA LAM to CUH 1960-10-7.

10. ANLMA Ex Comm NMA 1951-10-15.

11. ANLMA Report AGM 1964-06-04.

12. ANLMA AGM Resolutions 1958-05-04.

13. ANLMA AGM 1964-06-04.

14. ANLMA ARM to LAM 1963-01-31.

15. ANLMA LAM to ARM 1963-03-12.

16. ANLMA LAM to ARM 1963-04-08.

17. CNS JCCC LAM to JCC 1967-11-09.

18. CNS JCCC LAM to JCC 1968-03-04.

19. CNS JCCC LAM to JCC 1967-11-09.

20. CNS JCCC LAM to JCC 1968-03-04.

21. ANLMA Answers to Questions in House of Assembly, St. John's Daily News, 1960-04-04.

22. ANLMA AGM Minutes Resolution No. 13 1960-06-03.

23. ANLMA Ex Comm Meeting with J. McG and LAM 1960-7-29.

24. ANLMA ARM Report to AGM 1961-06-01-2-3 .

25. Royal Commission on Health, Right Honourable Lord Brain, January 1966. Published by Government of Newfoundland and Labrador. Recommendation 14.

26. NRC Miller Memoir (Unpublished).

27. The St. John's Evening Telegram 1963-11-19.

28. ANLMA The Newfoundland Medical Association Press Release 1963 - 11-21.

29. ANLMA First Draft for NMA Newsletter l963-12-31

30. ANLMA Ex Comm NMA 1963-11-13 .

31. ANLMA Ex Comm NMA 1963-11-17.

32. ANLMA WPC to PW 1963-10-18.

33. ANLMA Colonial Broadcasting Company Radio Station Marystown 1963-11-08.

34. ANLMA Special Note Secretary 1963-11-18 .

35. ANLMA Ex Comm. 1963-11-14.

36. ANLMA J McG to EP 1963-11-21.

37. ANLMA EJP to EP 1963-12-13.

38. ANLMA DH to NMA 1964-01-10.

39. ANLMA Ex Comm 1963-11-20.

CHAPTER 18

Occupational Health

Miller's education lay in classical Public Health, when occupational health was in its infancy. After World War II, occupational health made great strides. How well he kept abreast of these advances is a moot point. Still, his administrative duties also included occupational health, and during his term of office he was called upon to cope with one occupational health disaster of major proportions – the epidemic of radiation-induced cancer of the lungs at St. Lawrence.

In his day the only industrial activities of any significance in the province were several paper and pulp plants, a few mines and Smallwood's short-lasting industries. It was to the mines that Miller had to give most attention. The Mines Safety of Workers Act of 1951 split occupational health between the Department of Health and the Department of Mines, Agriculture and Resources (MAR).

On the whole, the two departments cooperated reasonably amicably in discharging their responsibilities in workers' health, but the following incident illustrates the very different philosophies that the two held about the role of the Department of Health in workers' health.

A worker wrote to the Federal Department of NH&W complaining of dust conditions in his workplace. The Minister sent a copy of his letter to Miller who without consulting with MAR, hired an outside specialist to conduct an on-site investigation of dust conditions in the mining operations. He confirmed that levels were high, due to inefficient exhaust ventilation and recommended remedial measures.[1] The Department of Health sent a copy of his report to MAR and to the offending company. In the letter to the company the Department of Health indicated its agreement with the specialist's report and requested the company to specify what corrective measures it would take.[2] In its acknowledgment of this letter, the company stated that it had already acted on the outside specialist's recommendations and had produced "very substantial improvement in dust conditions" and that the problem would soon "be solved to everybody's satisfaction."[3] In his letter the Minister of Health had told the company that its Chief Health Inspector would be visiting the mine soon to check on dust levels. The Department was obviously concerned about the danger of pneumoconiosis in this mine, fears that unfortunately later were proved to be only too well founded.[4] The Minister asked Miller if he had the authority to order the company to implement corrective measures.[5] Miller minuted "yes."

This incident brings out the dilemma facing a government department when it was suspicious that all was not well. To have closed down the operations until dust levels were satisfactory would have been to court economic ruin for the workers. Rightly or wrongly, the Department elected to accept management's assurances that the problem was coming under control. MAR, understandably, was put out by the steps taken by the Department of Health unilaterally in response to the worker's complaint.[6] In his acknowledgment of receipt of the outside specialist's report and the Department's letter to the company, the Minister of MAR quite properly questioned the need to hire an outside specialist to survey dust conditions because, he wrote, his department had the qualified staff to do this. He went on to say that his department had been concerned with dust levels in this mining operation since its inception, yet "the records show that steady improvements have been made towards reducing the concentration of dust." The Minister then made these extraordinary statements: "Although dust concentrations are above the permissible levels most of the time, employees are rotated in and out of these conditions in such a way that it is believed their health is not impaired." The Minister concluded by suggesting that "the

Department of Health should withdraw from direct intervention in this matter because if it does not there will be a divided responsibility for the enforcement of dust suppression measures . . . I would suggest that the proper function and responsibility of the Department of Health in connection with the operations of this plant in the future, [is] that whenever a medical examiner finds . . . that the health of an employee was being jeopardized would be to inform the mine inspectors so that drastic steps can be immediately taken." In other words, the Minister of MAR was limiting the role of the Department of Health to the detection of occupational diseases not their prevention. In commenting on this letter, Miller pointed out to the Minister of Health that he had "an overriding authority and in fact obligation . . . to prevent and to remedy conditions hazardous to health." Always conciliatory, Miller thought that both departments could carry out their duties without getting in each other's way.[7] Unfortunately, the exchange doesn't bear out his optimism. As shall be shown later, it was already becoming apparent at St. Lawrence that failure of the two departments to work together when a crisis developed could have serious consequences.

Even in environmental health Miller had to fight to preserve an active and decisive role for the Department of Health. In response to a proposal to transfer responsibility to MAR for "Prevention and Abatement for Environmental Health problems," Miller expressed his opposition. "This is so obviously a function of the Department of Health (if taken, an entirely new attitude towards prevention and control of disease in man would have to be developed), perhaps this is what is intended, but I find it hard to believe."[8]

Looking back one can see that occupational health can be planned effectively only if all parties to its enforcement see its role primarily as prevention not detection of disease. This could come about only by giving it independent status by creating a Division of Occupational Health and Safety, something which would have to wait until the St. Lawrence tragedy was played out and Miller had retired.

St. Lawrence

No field of medicine is more subject to public pressures than occupational health. Whenever there is an outbreak of an occupationally-related disease among the workers of an industry, the rest of the community and the media are drawn in and pressures are brought to bear on the authorities to take action. No government can afford to ignore such an outcry. At all costs it must give the impression that it is taking the community's concerns seriously and doing everything in its power to get to the root of the problem and identify those responsible for being negligent. In such an emotionally charged atmosphere, judicious, dispassionate decisions are not easy. These sentences summarize the events that unfolded at the St. Lawrence fluorspar mines in the middle third of this century. On the shoulders of the departments of health and MAR, fell the business of dealing with the tragedy, for such it proved to be.* How competently and with what sensitivity did they handle their tasks and how should Miller's performance be rated? An account of what happened should provide the answers to these and other questions.

Fluorspar Mining began at St. Lawrence in 1933. After World War II a widespread unease began to spread through the community. Chest complaints were common amongst the miners and some patients did not seem to respond to treatment but wasted away and died.[9] The MHO in the area was concerned and in 1950 asked the federal department of NH&W to undertake a dust and health survey.** He was told that the department could do so only if invited by the Newfoundland Department of Health. He does not appear to have made any further moves, but by 1953 the department of MAR had also become concerned and carried out its own dust survey. Fears were expressed that silicosis might be the explanation for the miners chest complaints. MAR arranged a conference with the Department of Health and the Workmen's Compensation Board at which Miller represented the Department of Health. The conference recommended that ambient dust and epidemiological studies should be undertaken. The results of these investigations were reported at another joint conference in 1954. They showed an increased incidence of tuberculosis and a few cases of silicosis, but surprisingly the dust levels were not above the then legally permissible and presumed safe levels for workers exposed to silica-containing dust.[10] In May 1955 another conference was held of the same

* For extensive accounts of the calamity see Leyton E. *Dying hard. The ravages of industrial carnage* and Adams, Ian, *The Poverty Wall.*

** It is not recorded whether this was verbally or in writing.

parties and experts on silicosis from Ontario. The purpose was to draft stricter regulations to prevent silicosis since this was assumed to be the problem. Dr. F. Brent, the Chief Medical Officer of The Aluminum Company of Canada (Alcan), the owner of the mines, must also have been present at this conference for he recalled "Dr. Miller was interested in getting to the bottom of this thing and I know that when the dust results came out and they didn't show anything significant, he was still very much in a quandary." [11]

At this point a startling development occurred. In 1954, Dr. C.J. Walsh, had come as MHO to the recently opened St. Lawrence Cottage Hospital.* He showed that the high death rate among the miners was in part due to cancer of the lungs. He identified 11 deaths between 1949 and 1955, statistically a significant increase. He brought his findings to the attention of the Department of Health and Dr. Brent. Everyone was puzzled because geiger counter checks of the mines in 1952-53 had not shown raised radiation levels. In 1956 MAR approached the federal department of NH & W requesting a survey of dust and health conditions to confirm that dust levels were normal. Once again the department of MAR was told that the federal authorities could act only in response to an invitation from the provincial Department of Health. It is not recorded when the official invitation was issued, but studies on dust conditions were being conducted by the Industrial Hygiene Division of NH & W in late 1956, and in 1958 these were expanded to include epidemiologic studies. The epidemiologic studies confirmed the presence of a high incidence of carcinoma of the lung.[12]

It was assumed by those conducting the survey that the miners were inhaling a carcinogenic dust, and over a year was spent in fruitless testing of mine dust for carcinogenicity. It was only in 1959 (at the suggestion of Brent) that attention was directed to an examination for radiation . The search was concluded when very high levels of radiation were found in unused and unventilated tunnels, and less high in working tunnels. The explanation was that although background radiation in the granite bedrock containing the veins of fluorspar was high, it presented no public danger because it escaped into the atmosphere. However, radon daughters were diffusing into

* A gift from the President of the USA in gratitude for the rescue operations mounted by the people of the region when two US destroyers ran aground in 1942. Miller used to argue that there were more practical ways of expressing appreciation than in constructing one more hospital in a region that already had two.

water in cracks in the bedrock, then entering the ground water and from thence seeping into the mine, where because of inadequate of ventilation, their concentration rose to hazardous levels. Installation of an efficient exhaust system brought the levels of radiation down to safe background levels.

Unfortunately, this did not help those who had been fatally exposed and who later were to develop cancer of the lungs. Workmen's compensation legislation had to be amended to make cancer of the lungs a compensable condition. But this did not allay the seething discontent in the community at what was seen as the delay in finding the cause, nor in settling the amount and procedures for compensation as well as entitlement; for it was argued that miners who contracted chronic bronchitis, emphysema and tuberculosis should also be entitled to compensation.[13, 14] Well aware that community resentments were smouldering, Smallwood appointed a Royal Commission in 1967 to report "on radiation , compensation and safety at the fluorspar mines in St. Lawrence." The Commission presented its findings in 1969.[9] Two of its conclusions and recommendations relate to the Newfoundland Department of Health.

The Department, and by implication this meant Miller, was censured " for being unduly slow in its acknowledgments of serious occupational hazards in the mines at St. Lawrence." There is nothing in the transcript of the Royal Commission to indicate that the Department was questioned by the Commission nor given an opportunity to defend itself. The sequence of response reactions as related above hardly supports the censure. It was realized by 1956 that the province was facing an outbreak of occupation-induced lung cancer and investigations to find the cause had been started right away. Two years later epidemiologic studies to confirm what was already known were initiated. It's hard to accuse Miller of procrastination in tackling the disaster. However, the Royal Commission rightly recognized that the operations of occupational health were hampered by its distribution between two departments, and recommended a separate division of industrial health within the Department of Health. The creation of the new division was implemented after Miller's retirement but it was placed in the Department of Labour. Looking back it is surprising that Miller never seems to have referred to the draw-back of divided responsibility for occupational health or to the obvious solution.

In the face of a catastrophe of such proportions, it was understandable to look for culprits to blame. The blanket condemnation of the Department of Health may have gone somewhat towards satisfying these expectations. In fact, the censure had no impact on the Department which, according to the recollections of a former Minister of Health, understood the Royal Commission's mandate as extending only to compensation. Accordingly, it took no notice of the reprimand nor took any measures to defend itself.

The rebuke cast no cloud over Miller's later career. He continued to enjoy the confidence and esteem of his Minister and Smallwood up to his retirement two years later.

The accusation has been made that Miller was not too interested in occupational health. Certainly it was not his major interest. On the other hand, whenever an actual or potential occupational health problem was brought to his attention, the record shows he took prompt measures to deal with it. Furthermore, when an asbestos mine was opened at Baie Verte he and the Minister were concerned that there be efficient dust abatement procedures in place and close monitoring of the miners' health.

Chapter 18 – Notes

1. CNS JCCC Nelson HM *Report on Environmental Conditions at IOCC* 1968-02-13.

2. CNS JCCC JCC to CKH 1968-03-19.

3. CNS EMRC CKH to TAH 1968-5-30.

4. Martin JR, Muir DCF, Moore, E. et al *Pneumoconiosis in Iron Ore Surface Mining in Labrador*. Journal of Occupational Medicine. 30: 781-784 1988.

5. CNS JCCC JCC to LAM 1968-01-29.

6. CNS EMRC WRC to TAH 1968-07-24.

7. CNS EMRC LAM to TAH 1968 -08-24.

8. CNS EMRC LAM TO ER 1969-12-29.

9. Royal Commission Respecting Radiation, Compensation and Safety at the Fluorspar Mines at St. Lawrence, Newfoundland 1969. Printed by the Government of Newfoundland.

10. PANL Radiation II GN6 1967 J McG Press Release 1961- 03- 01.

11. PANL Radiation II GN6 1967.

12. DeVilliers AM Windlish JP *Lung Cancer in a Fluorspar Mining Community, Radiation Dust and Mortality Experience* British Journal of Industrial Medicine 21 (2) 94-109 1964.

13. Leyton, E. *Dying Hard. The Ravages of Industrial Carnage.* Toronto Mc Clelland and Stewart 1975. p. 14.

14. CNS HD 7916 N4 L49 Leyton E. *The Bureaucratisation of Anguish. The Workmen's Compensation Board in an Industrial Disaster.* 1977.

CHAPTER 19

Nursing

While Miller was deputy minister, there was lively debate on the type of training nursing students should receive as well as the expanding role of nurses. Where did his inclinations lie? Being a cautious man, he was careful not to commit himself, but he did express opinions on a number of points to the twofold debate.

He once said, "Since we face the continuing difficulty of finding enough professional people for the Health Field, it may be necessary to consider how certain work may best be done in other ways by other people."[1] Did he perhaps think of nurses doing jobs hitherto reserved for doctors? After all it was during his lifetime that nurses came to be recognized as more than obedient servants of physicians. He certainly didn't oppose the changing role of nurses, even if he did not enthusiastically go along with it. If he did not actively promote these new developments, it was because, like all reforms, he knew they brought in their wake new problems. Miller was very sensitive to the adverse consequences of what to others appeared to be nothing but improvements. His relations with the organized nursing profession illustrate his somewhat ambivalent views to changes that were coming anyway, but changes he hoped he could direct into desirable channels.

Shortage of nurses was to plague the province throughout Miller's career. The ratio of nurses to patients was the lowest in

Canada and on occasions the shortage led to bed closures.[2] Their salaries were usually the lowest in Canada.[3] Nurses began to be in a position to fight for their rights with the incorporation of the Association of Registered Nurses of Newfoundland (ARNN) in 1953.[4] Miller was supportive of this action, acting as advisor to the Association during the drafting of the Act of Incorporation. He assisted the Association in its continuing education programs by contributing to the expenses of visiting speakers. In the mid 1950s, the training of nursing students at the St. John's hospitals changed from the three year apprentice system to the " 2+1 system," that is, two years of instruction and one year of supervised experience on the wards.[5] To make up for the shortfall foreseen in personnel for bedside nursing due to this switch, a nursing assistant school was opened at the General Hospital. Miller saw the merit of these changes and was able to find the funding for the nursing assistant program.

In 1966, on its own initiative, MUN instituted a five year Bachelor of Nursing (BN) program. The first director, Ms. Joyce Nevitt, called on Miller shortly after her arrival to request government bursaries for students enrolled in the BN course and also for BN graduates who wished to obtain a postgraduate degree in some branch of nursing. At the time, the government awarded one year bursaries to registered nurses for postgraduate work on the Mainland. Miller refused to give bursaries for more than one year. She summed him up: "He was charming and gentle and easy to talk with, but you never quite knew where you stood with him. He was a politician and had to be cautious." The one year bursaries were popular with the local nurses wishing to do further studies and they didn't want to see any changes apart from having the opportunity of pursuing post graduate studies within the province. She left feeling that Miller sympathized with her request but was powerless to do anything about it. She could have been mistaken, as will become apparent.

Miller was cool to the MUN School of Nursing. He did not consciously mislead people, but he played his cards close to his chest. A frequent comment of those who had dealings with him was that you never knew what he was thinking, it was easy to come away from an interview believing whatever one wanted. For Miller, ever conscious of limited funds, it was the cost of any new venture which governed his attitude towards it. The MUN School of Nursing was funded out of education funds and therefore cost the Department of Health nothing, but Miller knew there would be a price to pay: a BN nurse would demand a higher salary than an RN.[6]

The BN program was the cause of another headache. Nursing students at the hospital-based nursing schools had free lodging and food, while the BN students were not so fortunate. Appeals were made to Miller to provide financial support for BN students. His reply was that they should not be treated differently than any other students and were he to give them financial assistance other health profession students would come asking for similar treatment.[7]

Miller's innate caution may be the reason that he never got involved in nurse-practitioner programs. To do so would have been to stir up hostilities in some medical quarters. On the other hand the Dalhousie Outpost Nursing Program in the IGA territory caused no ripples and could be tolerated since it was an arrangement between the IGA and Dalhousie University for the northern parts of the province only.

Miller's opinions on the practice of nursing and contemporary developments, come out in the report he submitted as a one man royal commissioner after his retirement.[8] Miller's mandate was "to make an inquiry into and concerning nursing education and regulations within the province." It was the first and only time he undertook a task of this nature. He certainly appears to have been thorough in his inquiries, but the report itself is somewhat too brief for a task of this nature and his recommendations were not helpful. At least he cannot be faulted for lack of diligence in soliciting submissions from those who had an interest in the training of nurses and in the regulation of the profession, and he certainly consulted the literature on the subject. He received twenty-four briefs one of which, from the ARNN, was presented at a public hearing. In his report, Miller commented on and criticized the briefs he had received, but omitted to reproduce any of them as appendices to his report. The reader therefore is unable to form any opinion of how fairly and thoroughly Miller dealt with each submission. Still, he does appear to have recognized one of the most significant questions facing hospital nursing schools, the dilemma of balancing education with service and avoiding the exploitation of student nurses as a pool of cheap labour. Although in recent years, he noted, there had been greater emphasis on education and reduction in ward drudgery, the ARNN and the MUN School of Nursing argued that the only way around this dilemma was to place the education component squarely in a University setting away from hospitals. This philosophy was beginning to reign in nursing circles but carried with it a price tag, as Miller realized. He noted that the hospital schools of nursing came under the Federal/Provincial Cost Share Programs on a per capita basis, and that in the province of Newfoundland the federal share was 60%. The MUN School of Nursing was also funded through a shared Federal/Provincial program, but came under postsecondary education grants. Were the province to eliminate hospital schools of nursing and expand the university school, it would obtain less funds on a per capita basis than it obtained under the Hospital Insurance and Diagnostic Services Acts. The difference in dollars would not be insignificant. Ever guided by financial considerations, Miller criticized the ARNN brief for ignoring this practical consideration.

Miller expressed his admiration for the thoroughness and persuasiveness of the submission from the MUN School of Nursing, but he concurred with the comments of the acting Dean of Arts under whom the school operated, that "measures for determining the quality of graduates have been notoriously poor." He expressed his concern at the evolution of the school, in particular its obsession with degrees. It offered only a Master's degree for post graduate studies, but would not provide what most Registered Nurses were able to afford, a one year diploma in a specialized course. Furthermore, he must have been skeptical of the benefit to the province of a school where almost all of the most recent graduating class had left the province.

Although aware of their deficiencies, Miller was more favourably inclined to the hospital nursing schools, probably because the length of training was less than at the university school and therefore less costly. He argued, perhaps somewhat optimistically, that in this setting "there should not have to be a conflict between nursing education and nursing service." He admitted that in spite of expansion of the education component of the training and curtailment of service "patient care still looms larger than it should." But he had come to the conclusion the hospital-based nursing schools could not continue as such, but would have to be relocated under "educational auspices".

When it came to making proposals Miller acknowledged "the lack of hard evidence on which to base recommendations; rather must they be based on recent and apparently successful experiments elsewhere, modified when necessary by local conditions." But Miller himself did not follow his own advice in presenting his recommendations. Instead of each recommendation flowing as a logical conclusion from a preceeding paragraph of narrative, providing the evidence to support it, his recommendations are tabulated early on in the report. They stand alone as expressions of personal opinion. This was another case where Miller's penchant for brevity did not stand him in good stead.

The most important recommendations relate to a nurse diploma course of "not longer than two years – within the general education system." Evidentally (Recommendation 2), he envisaged a College of Health Sciences or a College of Nursing for the St. John's hospital Nursing Schools, administered by the College of Trades and Technology. For the Western Memorial Hospital Nursing School at Corner Brook, he recommended joint operation by the Hospital Board and the Junior College of MUN.

The two year diploma course was championed by the spirit of the times and had received the endorsement of the Royal Commission on Health Services.[9] There were also those who advocated the transfer of nursing schools to junior colleges and Miller was only putting his seal of approval on what was occurring in other provinces. As should have been foreseen, the two year diploma courses were to prove a most unwise policy, since at graduation the students were found to be woefully deficient in practical experience. For this reason they were later dropped. Fortunately, the "2+1 system" survived in the province in spite of Miller's recommendation. One has no way of knowing whether Miller really believed in a two year diploma course or was going along with a trend in spite of misgivings.

No one would quarrel with his recommendation to make nurses' salaries more competitive with other provinces, since it was the financial attractions elsewhere which were responsible for the drainage of nurses from the province.

Miller had nothing to propose for the MUN School of Nursing except for the cryptic suggestion that it should "modify its policies with more emphasis on provincial needs." The most reasonable interpretation of this obscure piece of advice, seems to be that the school should enter the field of the one year postgraduate diploma courses.

While Miller was conducting his inquiry, the MUN School of Nursing initiated a pilot project to train registered nurses to fill an expanded role in urban centres in association with family practitioners that is, as nurse practitioners. Miller praised this project because of its "realistic process of evaluation", but nothing came of it.

The Royal Commission on Nursing Education met the same fate as many other Royal Commissions, to be put on a shelf and forgotten. Miller must share part of the blame for this outcome. Brevity was one of his virtues in daily administration but here it was a handicap. He had no innovative suggestions and his attitude to the BN program was backward even for those days. But perhaps his scepticism about the debate on nursing education comes out in his assessment of the nursing care he received during a period of hospitalization some time previously. He was careful to inquire about the educational background of each of the nurses who took care of him. There were BNs, RNs and graduates of the two year diploma courses. He said he could see no difference in the quality of nursing care each provided.[5]

On the whole, the Royal Commission on Nursing did not enhance Miller's reputation. He did not have the gift for this sort of work. His talents lay in exposing flaws in the work of others, as he so effectively succeeded in his critique of Lord Brain's report. But by the time he undertook the study on nursing his health had begun to fail.

Chapter 19 – Notes

1. Warrick, H.J. *Changing the Front Line of Community Health.* Newfoundland Medical Association Newsletter 11 (4): 8-11 1969.

2. CNS JCCC Nursing Situation in Newfoundland. Associadon of Registered Nurses Newfoundland memo 1967-12-20.

3. Association of Registered Nurses Brief to Royal Commission on Health 1966-01-2.

4. Story, J. Five Years of Progress. Canadian Nurse 55 (7):599-600 1959.

5. Story, J. Personal Communication.

6. CNS JCCC Association of Registered Nurses of Newfoundland Salary Brief 1966.

7. CNS JCCC LAM to JCC 1968-04-08.

8. *Royal Commission on Nursing Education.* Leonard A. Miller Commissioner, then Government of Newfoundland, February 1974.

9. Royal Commission on Health Services. Ottawa. Queen's Printer, 1964. Cat. no. Z1-1961/3-1 (Recommendation 127).

CHAPTER 20

Other Activities

Miller's duties and interests extended beyond the activities of physicians and nurses and their places of work. He was also responsible for the provision of dental services in the outports. From his earlier years he was active in health promotion, an interest he was to maintain throughout his career. Finally, like so many other administrators of his day, he depended on voluntary agencies to provide services outside the government's domain. No biography of Miller would be complete without taking some notice of his doings in these spheres.

Dental Services

Rural Newfoundland was no more able to support fee-for-service dentists than physicians. In 1950 there were only 19 dentists for the province, almost all in the larger centres.[1] Dental caries was rampant. Miller was quite convinced that one day it would come under control. Dr. David Peters, a dentist, remembers expressing his dismay about the extent of dental caries to Miller and receiving this reply: "Tuberculosis 20 years ago was a scourge, but look at today, only a few cases; likewise, dental caries will one day be under control." But to do so required a three-pronged approach.[2] First, prevention through fluoridation of water supplies. There were public concerns about the safety of this procedure which would have to be allayed before it could be introduced into a locality.[3] The second prong was education, and the third was provision of dental services.

The Children's Health Plan of 1955 provided for free dental services for children. The problem was the availability of dental services, especially in the Outports. It was even more difficult to attract dentists to remote areas than doctors. Smallwood of course had a simple solution to the dearth of dentists. "We're going to have fifty dentists come to Newfoundland even if we have to go behind the Iron Curtain to get them."[4] When the Newfoundland Dental Board, responsible for licensing, drew his attention to the requirement of establishing their proper qualifications before hiring them, Smallwood replied, "I will decide." He then proceeded to have the Dental Act amended, lowering qualifications for licensure. The upshot was that only a few overseas practitioners took the bait and most were so obviously incompetent that they had to be dismissed.[4]

How did one go about providing dental services in remote areas ? " It was a case of the chicken and the egg. Which came first? A demand for dental services or the provision of them, with the hope that they would then be utilized?"[4] Miller wisely decided it had to be both at the same time. Government-assisted dentists were recruited and located in areas where they could supplement their salaries through fee for service. After 1945, the government provided bursaries for Newfoundland dental students committed to returning and working in government-designated areas for specified periods.[5]

Health Education

The Department of PH&W of the Commission of Government was energetic in pursuing programs to educate the public in proper health practices. Miller was as enthusiastic in this respect as his predecessor, Mosdell. Even as an MHO he gave radio talks on current health problems. The government realized that the measure of a public health program was healthy children, and the key to its success was their teachers and public health nurses. For some years Miller gave a course on preventive medicine to student teachers at Memorial College. Until 1949, the government was also active assisting in the formation of branches of the Junior Red Cross in schools as a means of spreading information on good health practices. One of the last acts of the Commission of Government was to commission a health education survey by Margaret E. Nix under the auspices of the PH&W Department.[6]

Nix recommended the establishment of a division to coordinate health education programs and to conduct in- service training of all public health and welfare staff. Daphne Pratt (later House), who had been working in Health Education for the Department, was appointed Director.[7] She had been trained in education and was able to bring innovative and up-to-date ideas and methods for putting the message across. She acknowledged her indebtedness to Miller for making her understand that she could only work successfully through the teachers, public health nurses, and nutritionists. Miller was, she describes, "a most kind and considerate boss, full of sage advice." When she was saddled with the responsibility of illness in her family, he arranged flexible working hours for her.

Voluntary Agencies

In a country with as few financial resources as Newfoundland, private initiative had to supplement or supply services which the government could not afford. In the Health Survey of 1956 Miller acknowledged government's indebtedness to a number of these voluntary agencies.[1] The one that was probably closest to his heart was the Child Welfare Association, founded in 1920 by a group of benevolent ladies. It ran children's health and maternal clinics in St. John's, staffed by nurses and volunteers. Evaporated milk, cod liver oil and later concentrated orange juice were distributed free of charge in those days of wide-spread poverty and malnutrition. Miller took a great interest in the clinics and attended them until he became DMS. His tact, skill and sympathy in handling mothers and children were legendary. A volunteer remembers vividly the day Miller noticed a mother was still clasping her dead baby. Miller quietly went over and put a comforting arm around her.[8]

Miller started welfare clinics in neighbouring communities close to St. John's, but such was the spirit of the times that there had to be separate clinics for Protestants and Roman Catholics![8]

Nobody could describe these Outport clinics as dull. When Miller and his staff arrived the start of the clinic had to be announced. In one Outport, like a town crier of times gone by, a volunteer would go to a nearby church and ring the bell to tell all and sundry that the clinic had opened its doors.[8] Miller had to be satisfied with whatever premises were put at his disposal. Usually it was a hall. He had to be ready for the unexpected. On one occasion the holding of a child welfare clinic was delayed until a hearse could be removed from the premises.[8]

Chapter 20 – Notes

1. CNS RA450N4, N36 Newfoundland. Health Survey Committee. Newfoundland Health Survey Report . Chairperson L.A. Miller 1956.

2. PANL Health Dental Box 9361 LAM to HJH 1958 -04 -12.

3. PANL Health Dental Box 9361 LAM to WAP 1965 -05-23.

4. Peters, D. Personal Communication.

5. Miller, L *Placement Incentives*: (Letter) Canadian Medical Association Journal 126 (2): 120 1982.

6. PANL GN 26/7/3 *Newfoundland Department of Public Health & Welfare. Education Survey*. Margaret Nix 1949.

7. Pratt, Daphne, *Public Health Education in Newfoundland*. Canadian Journal Public Health 48:153-7 1957.

8. Ayre, Olga Personal Communication.

CHAPTER 21

The Department of Health

During Miller's day, the Department of Health was able to make decisions much more rapidly than under his successors. There were no cabinet committees nor requirements for approval at multiple levels. Consequently, business could be dispatched expeditiously. In such a system, a Deputy Minister who had been around as long as Miller, came to exercise considerable power. Miller tended to put little in writing but to carry the most detailed knowledge about a question in his head. Yet it was obvious in discussion that he had all the information at his fingertips. Furthermore, in keeping with his ways of doing things, departmental meetings were kept informal.

Miller was the chief civil servant in the Department of Health for twenty-seven years. He never became arrogant but remained self-effacing and conciliatory to the end of his career. There is no record of a Minister reining him in, but it has been said that sometimes he would venture too far and be cautioned; then all he would do would be to give his famous smile. His ways for transacting business were often informal. On one occasion at midnight after a long day, out of the blue he said to two of his staff, "This is a good time to have a planning session over a bottle of Screech.* We'll let our hair down and see what ideas we can come up with to improve the health care system." Sure enough, according to one of the two, they did come up with some bright ideas, several of which were later implemented.

*A popular drink in Newfoundland, distilled from the washings from rum barrels.

His ways for reaching agreement could be unorthodox. A decision was urgently required on the salary scale for a group of health workers. Miller's solution was to take two of his assistants into a room. "I'm disconnecting the phone. We can't leave here until we've decided what they are going to get next year." A decision was reached. Miller wrote the proposed salary scale on a piece of paper and then took it over to the Deputy Minister of Finance, who after grumbling "where's the money to come from?" initialled the proposal. Miller then got on the telephone and told the head of the health worker's association of the decision and the next day the Minister announced the new salary scale in the Legislature. Nowadays there would have been some hard bargaining with union representatives. The only dealings Miller had with this group was the brief it sent him setting out its case for a salary increase.

To the extent that he had a free hand, Miller's aim was to surround himself with a staff in whom he had confidence and could trust. One official recalls being approached by Miller and told to apply for a particular position. She argued that S was more qualified. Miller replied, "I'm not asking S to apply, it is you that I'm asking." No wonder those whom Miller chose should almost idolize him. He expected them to be as single-minded and hard working as he was and they rose to the challenge. Because Miller sought to choose his own staff he has been accused of favouritism, but there was nothing to suggest that his choice was dictated by anything else than of a person's ability to perform the task he had in mind and to work harmoniously with others. As the years went by, he gathered around himself a support staff he had trained and in whom he had confidence. He would call them together every few weeks to discuss what was going on in the department. Miller had the great virtue of being able to delegate and to give those who worked under him a free hand. He had a good grasp of the financial resources available to him and was a master at juggling his budget to find money for a new project. Nevertheless, he preferred to delegate budgeting to T. Sellars, one of the administrative officers in the department, and to concentrate his energies on policy and dealing with people.

In administrative matters he sought to keep things simple. "All that I am trying to do is to see if we can cut down the amount of paper work."[1] He was not always successful. A former superintendent of nurses at the General Hospital recalls her frustration at the amount of red tape she had to go through to get permission for leave of absence.

Anyone bringing a proposition to Miller had to satisfy him that there was a clear reason for the proposal. He had no time for high sounding phrases such as, "it would be better for the health of the province etc." This line would be quikly interrupted with "yes, yes, we've heard all that before," and Miller would put his three basic questions: "Why do you want this? Who is going to benefit by it? How is it going to solve the problem?" Unless Miller's demands on these three points were satisfied and he was convinced of the utility of the proposal, the caller could not hope for a sympathetic hearing. Once convinced, he would support a proposal through thick and thin and go to no end of trouble to find the funds for its implementation.

One of Miller's greatest assets was his imperturbability. During his years as Deputy Minister he had reason to call on it frequently. The Smallwood era has been likened to government by crisis. No one knew what he might be up to next, what impossible situation into which he might suddenly land himself and the government. His officials would be aghast on these occasions, wondering how they could extricate themselves and him from some appalling situation. But Miller, throughout the storm, would remain serene, calm and unruffled, a general steadying his troops. A government official

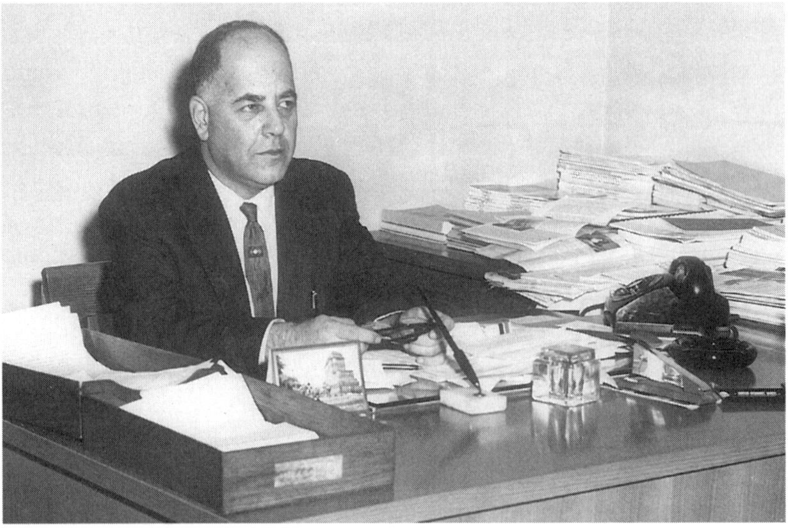

The Deputy Minister of Health at his desk. Courtesy Mrs. L. Balderson

remembers expressing his dismay about one of Smallwood's escapades, exclaiming that there was no possible way out of the disaster. "Don't worry", said Miller. "Wait a while, we will get all that sorted out." Sure enough he was right as in the days that followed he quietly initiated damage control. To be able to roll with the punches was a great asset in those days.

Miller managed his staff with great skill. No one complained of intimidation. He rarely issued orders and then only in the most urgent circumstances. He preferred to work by persuasion, asking and suggesting. But when action was required, he would call his staff together, discuss what needed to be done, listen to their opinions and involve them in the final decision. The staff remembers that he was always in control of the discussion. His was leadership of the highest order and it is easy to see why those who worked under him look back to those days with nostalgia: "He lead by example, by suggestion, by support and by quiet collegial discussion, especially when we did something unwisely."

His staff enjoyed bringing their problems to him, sitting down and discussing them with him. "He would bring out aspects that had escaped my notice and if I said something foolish he would floor me with a smile." One functionary recalls taking her problem to Miller who, after listening, assured her she didn't have one. She expostulated that she did, but back came the answer, "No you don't, for every problem there is a solution." In other words what could not be cured had to be endured.

Unlike many administrators, he did not leave interpersonal conflicts to solve themselves. An official complained to Miller of rudeness from a colleague. Miller called both into his office, listened to each of their views, made his own comments and got both of them to shake hands.

Since Miller was responsible for the day-to-day administration of the Department, it followed that he should accept blame for the actions of his subordinates. He was punctilious in doing so and never protected himself at their expense.

There was one thing however that roused Miller to decisive action – a misdemeanor of an employee. The Department had collected evidence that a Cottage Hospital employee was stealing government supplies. The official in the department to whom the employee was responsible mentioned to Miller that he was about to set out on a tour of a number of Cottage Hospitals and would drop in on the culprit's hospital on his way back and deal with the case. "Drop in first at that hospital right away and investigate his case," said Miller in peremptory terms that brooked no contradiction nor delay. He did so and found enough evidence to justify dismissal of the employee on the spot. On another occasion, a senior official in the Department was suspected of pocketing government money. Miller made sure of his facts and then called the accused into his office. The latter denied any wrong doing. "You are a good liar, but I will prove what you have done," said Miller in cold, and firm tones. He did so and the official was sent packing.

Miller's low key personality had no quirks or foibles for his subordinates to poke fun at. The one exception was his deep voice. Several employee's in the department learned to mimic it to perfection and would telephone other employees, and amuse themselves at their expense. One staff member recalls receiving a call at his house and assuming it was from one of the pranksters, answered in bantering terms. After a few minutes he realized to his horror that it was the real Dr. Miller speaking to him. He extricated himself as well as he could under the circumstances. The next day when he reported to Miller no reference was made to his egregious behaviour. "It was as if it had never occurred."

Every day a stream of visitors would pass through Miller's office. Doctors posted to a Cottage Hospital or a rural district would report for briefing before proceeding . They would also drop in with complaints. Whatever the reason for their visits, they would often come out looking happier than when they went in, so adept was Miller at smoothing ruffled feathers and dissipating complaints. Miller encouraged salaried physicians to call him or to drop in at his office and if he could not see them then, he would give them an appointment to come back.

How did Miller appear from the other side of the desk? What first caught the eye, was the high dome-shaped forehead. It was even more striking in his younger days when he had a thatch of hair on top of it . But then as he began to speak, it was the famous smile which captured attention. Like a beacon, it flashed on and off. "A Mona Lisa smile," says one caller. Another, a "Sphinx-like smile." As the smile came and went, the visitor could not help wondering if it signified approval or disapproval. Perhaps Miller intended to leave his visitor guessing.

When the topic to be discussed was pleasant, Miller would appear affable and easy going. At other times, you realized the smile masked a very different person who could be quite forceful when needed. But he preferred not to conduct his business this way. In discussion he would lead the caller, have him come up with the options and his preference. If Miller then approved, he would endorse it.

Because Miller was so careful in phrasing his opinions he has been accused of never making a definite statement. A colleague grumbled that the only positive statement he had ever made was at his daughter's wedding in response to the clergyman's inquiry, "Who giveth this woman in marriage?" But those who worked with him knew that, like all wise politicians, he avoided making rash promises and sought to keep his options open as long as he could. But when the time came that a commitment had to be made, he did not hesitate to do so and then to stick to it. Miller was skilled at calming people down by a funny comment or some other action to defuse the situation. He was equally versatile when it came to deflecting complaints. A delegation from the outports called on Miller complaining of the life-style of their physician. They left his office fully persuaded they were getting excellent health care, which was the important thing, never mind the doctor's eccentricities.

Sometimes loud voices were heard from his office but they never came from Miller. There was only one official in his department with whom he sometimes had heated arguments, but they never degenerated into shouting matches. Miller's office was separated from the Minister's by a room which served as common waiting room and office for the secretaries. This made it easy for the Minister and Deputy Minister to drop in on each other .

Miller attached great importance to his informal talks with the Minister over a cup of tea. He wisely believed the Department must never admit the services it provided were deficient – stretched, perhaps, but never inadequate or below par. A Minister, in a draft reply to a patient's complaint about the medical services he had received, had written, "Again I realize that this service is far from perfect, but again it is the best we can do with the means at our disposal etc."[2] This was an inadmissable excuse in Miller's eyes and he advised its deletion and replacement by these high sounding phrases which eschewed apology for unsatisfactory services: "I realize that we shall never be able to have doctors and nurses available every time anybody is sick. I am sure, however, that with your cooperation as well as that of other interested citizens, our people will receive the best services possible in the circumstances."

Miller and His Secretaries

A gentleman, so it is said, is not a hero to his valet. No words could be further from the truth in the case of Miller and his secretaries. It says much that from 1948 to 1968 he had only two secretaries and each speaks of him in glowing terms. One, sending him a gift after her retirement, summed up her feelings in these words: "They [cuff links] carry with them from me the most pleasant memories of a type of association that is given to few. I realize my good fortune and thank you for everything." In their eyes he was thoughtful and considerate. The father of one of his secretaries died. She had never told Miller but was surprised to see him at the funeral. Another departmental secretary who had reached the top of the salary scale for her classification, was advised by Miller to apply for the job of secretary to the Minister because it carried with it a higher salary. Relunctantly she followed his advice. Both the long term secretaries said he brought out the best in them. He was discriminating in praise but knew when to show appreciation as in the following letter to one of his secretaries upon her retirement: "Your continuous presence during the most difficult years made a vast difference to me and my work. I shall always remember your . . . willing assistance and the high quality of your work."

To his secretaries Miller was an example for senior officials to emulate. He was a man of few words, a ready listener presenting a calm, unruffled front to his staff. He knew when the time had come to make a decision, but did so only after carefully weighing the facts and, if circumstances allowed, sitting on it for a couple of days. When an unpalatable decision had to be broken to someone, Miller did not shirk from doing it himself. Towards the end of his career, it was imperative an experienced secretary be brought in to prepare for his successor. Miller insisted it was his responsibility to break the news to his current secretary of her impending displacement. Miller observed a strict etiquette in his office. He always appeared in a shirt and tie; and in front of others, secretaries were always addressed by their surnames prefixed by Mrs. or Miss. Business was transacted only in the office, never in the corridor.

A typical office day began at 9:00 a.m. with Miller's arrival. He first attended to his mail and went over matters that required a decision. When he was ready he would call in his secretary for dictation. He never used a dictaphone. Each letter or item requiring a memo would be taken up in turn and slowly, without notes or changes, Miller would dictate. His dictation flowed like a stream. If he was interrupted he would have the last sentence repeated and then take up from there. When the secretary brought back letters and memoranda for his signature, the only changes that he made would be corrections of her typographical errors.

At one time it was the custom to put copies of the past week's non-confidential departmental correspondence on display in a reading room of the department. Miller's correspondence used to attract the most notice. It was a model of brevity. He himself detested long letters and would have agreed with the writer who apologized for a long letter because he didn't have time to write a shorter one. A typical Miller letter or memorandum would be two or three pages, double spaced. The relevant points would be tabulated. If it was a memorandum to the Minister, Miller would wisely, enumerate the possible responses or actions and leave it to the Minister to make his own choice. But if there was a particular choice which Miller did not want the Minister to make he would give the reasons against it. Miller was well aware a Minister has a name to make for himself and must believe that he is formulating policy and is not the pawn of the Deputy Minister. However, his memoranda are not always free from grammatical errors and he did not always make his meaning clear.

If the telephone rang while Miller was dictating, he himself would answer it. He disliked long telephone calls. At Miller's end of the telephone, silences were punctuated by grunts or a 'yes' or a 'no.' One conversation ended with the advice, " You can do one of two things, and one of them is nothing." A physician who had frequent dealings with Miller likened him on the telephone to a telegram with no prepositions or articles, just a series of nouns and verbs strung together.

Miller's secretaries were expected to attend to his creature comforts by supplying midmorning tea and purchasing his cigarettes. At one time he was a heavy smoker, but rarely finished a cigarette. Suddenly, in the mid 1960s he stopped, wrote the date of his salvation on the last empty package and kept it for years as a memento.

On the wall of his office was a map of Newfoundland with the Cottage Hospitals flagged as well as the names of the current Cottage Hospital doctors. The other item of interest on the wall was a graph of infant mortality in the province. Each year a new dot was added and a line drawn between it and the previous one. For Miller, infant mortality was the best indicator of a nation's health.

Gender Issues

Nowadays people would want to know where the subject of a biography stood when it came to the treatment of women. Miller has been praised for promoting women such as Daphne House to the key position of the Director of Health Education. Women who worked for him have nothing but the highest praise for his fairness in employment practices. Payment however, was a different matter. In the first decade after Confederation female doctors in the sanatoria were paid less than men for the same position.* [3] But by 1961 employees of both sexes were paid according to "authorized salary scales." [4] In theory discrimination had ended. But overt discrimination in the government services continued to exist for some years, in the provision for the compulsory retirement of a female civil servant upon marriage, unless the Minister recommended retention, and then it could only be on a temporary basis. At least, where he could, Miller promoted the employment of women to responsible positions. But he does not seem to have deprecated the inequality of pay . He could have defended himself by arguing that with a limited budget he had no choice but to purchase services as cheaply as possible. Why should he pay an employee more than he had to?

* In Miller's day, salaried female physicians were rare. I can find no reference to their presence in the cottage hospital scheme before Confederation. After 1949 there were several husband and wife teams and the occasional female physician. However, there were several salaried female physicians in the sanatoria both before and after 1949.

Miller's informal ways of transacting business, putting little in writing but relying on his phenomenal memory, became a matter of concern as his retirement drew closer. Fears were expressed that this did not allow for a smooth transfer of power and his successor would find himself coping with matters about which he was in the dark. Miller's ways began to be labelled archaic. The management firm KPM which had been retained in 1967 to advise on the implementation of medicare warned that management practices and organization would have to change to meet new conditions.[5] The firm's mandate was extended to examine the administrative structures of the Department and to make recommendations. A more "collegial" way of arriving at decisions was recommended with less authority resting in the hands of the Deputy Minister. These changes were introduced after Miller's retirement but not to the satisfaction of all the staff in the department. One senior official told me he left in frustration at the slowness of getting things done under the new regime. Another recalls that after Miller left, things "weren't the same. Everything became much more bureaucratic."

Chapter 21 – Notes

1. CNS Box 9363 Health Department LAM to DGB-W 1962-04-26.

2. CNS EMRC LAM to ER 1970-2-20.

3. CNS JRSC JMcG Memo 1956-07-12.

4. CNS JRSC JMcG Memo 1961-03-06, 1961-07-05.

5. CNS JCCC RAD to JCC1968-04-10,and 1968-04-11.

CHAPTER 22

The Cabinet

When Miller became a full-time employee of the government in 1934, the Commissioner of the PH&W and Welfare was John C. Puddester with Dr. H.M. Mosdell as his secretary. In his memoir, Miller has the highest praise for both these men and the debt Newfoundland owes to them but says nothing about his working relations with them.[1] In 1944 when Mosdell died, Miller was assigned the health part of his job, except for the St. John's hospitals, with the title Director of Medical Services. Later he became responsible for the St. John's hospitals also. Then in 1947, Sir John Puddester died and was succeeded by H.W. Quinton, who was in ill health for most of the time. He also served as Minister of Health for the first few months of the Smallwood government and then was replaced by J.R. Chalker.

When Newfoundland joined Confederation, Miller realized that he was entering an entirely new world. Shortly after he was appointed Deputy Minister he told Chalker, "There are going to be lots of changes. For the first time in my life I'm going to be working with a government that runs its institutions to get votes. Before you make any changes please let me know." Chalker was happy to give this commitment, but in return said to Miller, "Advise me, don't go over my head to Smallwood." Miller's reply was, "If I want anything, I will go to you and take my orders from you." Both men stuck to their bargain. Thus from the very beginning they were able to establish workable and cordial relations. Chalker did not pretend to know anything about health and was quite happy to be guided by Miller and to let him run the department. "I was fortunate to have him as my Deputy. " Miller for his part had little to say about the first three Ministers of Health after Confederation, except to write that relations were smooth and that they left him to run the department and sometimes even to write their speeches.[1] In 1956 a much more intimate partnership between Minister and Deputy Minister was to develop. Dr. James McGrath (1902-75), who had been Miller's assistant since 1944, was persuaded by Smallwood to run for the legislature with the intimation that if elected he would be given a Cabinet post. McGrath was elected and was promptly appointed Minister of Health.

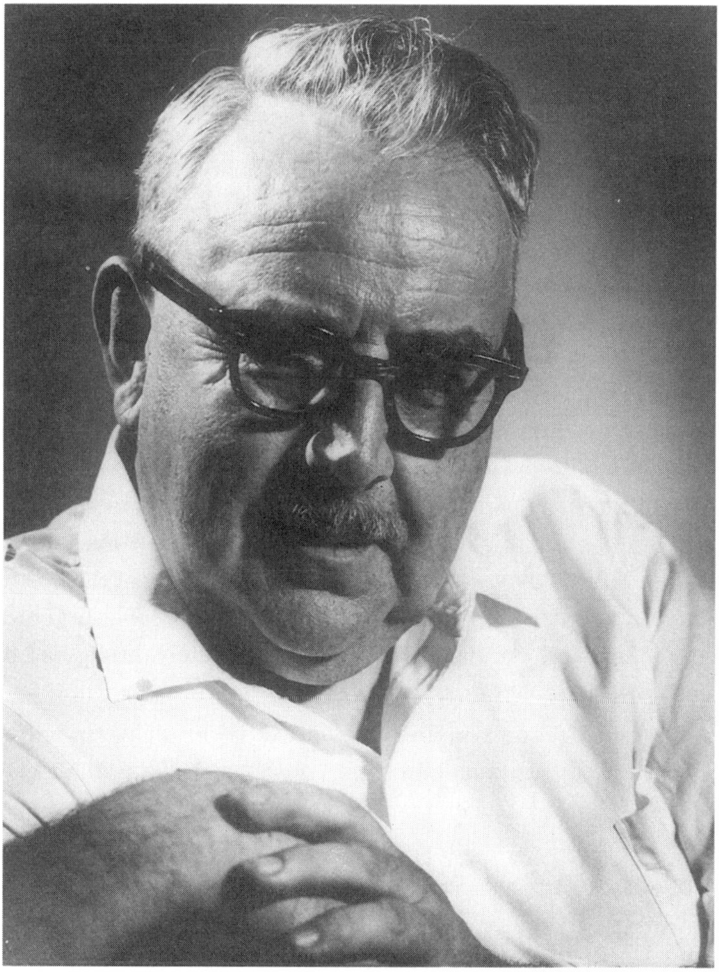

Dr. James McGrath *Courtesy Mrs. Janet Kelly*

McGrath came from a prominent Newfoundland family. He was a man of many talents – a voracious reader and a poet; a fluent and witty speaker. He would while away the tedium of sittings of the Legislature by reading French poetry or novels. He was a few years older than Miller and became an MHO about the same time as Miller. Like Miller, he had been in private practice[2] and then had taken post-graduate studies in public health. However, Miller had got a start on McGrath in the ranks of the civil service and McGrath could not hope to pull ahead if he had continued as a government employee. In a sense they should have been rivals but instead a firm friendship developed between the two men. In 1944 he became Miller's deputy and remained so until his elevation to Minister. He had been the government official responsible for directing, very competently, the campaign against tuberculosis, but by the time he had attained Cabinet rank, it was obvious that tuberculosis was coming under control. He would need some new field in which to display his talents. The McGrath and Miller families had been friends for many years. A McGrath daughter recalls Miller playing with the McGrath children, dangling them by their legs and dropping his partial plate to the amusement of the children, if not of Myra. The McGrath children loved him and felt completely at ease in his company. McGrath and Miller had discussed Smallwood's invitation and agreed that if McGrath obtained a seat in the Cabinet he would then have the political clout to push through measures that they both thought desirable. The reversal of their roles did not effect their friendship in the least.* Their attitude was that a job had to be done and the person best qualified should be the one delegated to do it. It was obvious to both of them that Miller's talents did not lie in the hurly-burly of the hustings. McGrath told a daughter that Miller "was utterly reliable, and utterly honest". The two men trusted each other completely throughout their careers; a period of unbroken friendship.

One could not imagine two more different personalities. McGrath was gregarious, bluff and impatient. Unlike Miller he did not take the trouble to be punctiliously courteous with subordinates or to cultivate good relations with them. One who held a junior post in the department describes him as "arrogant, bombastic, irascible

* The story of their relationship would be incomplete without reference to a rumor that it was in order to leapfrog over Miller that McGrath had entered politics. There is nothing to substantiate that this was his motivation.

and abrupt, with no social graces. If Miller passed you in the hall he always smiled at you while McGrath would walk right past you as if he had never seen you. He wouldn't hesitate to dress you down in front of others, something Miller would never do." McGrath could also be guilty of hasty decisions and, unlike Miller, frequently rubbed people the wrong way. These were to prove serious handicaps in his relations with the NMA, and were flaws in a man with otherwise many brilliant and fine qualities, admired and respected by Miller and a large circle of friends.

If McGrath was a novice when he joined the Cabinet, he quickly learned the tricks of the trade. He became notorious for finding positions for young people from his constituency at the government hospitals.

Miller put his finger on one of McGrath's serious weaknesses. McGrath could be high-handed in his disputes with the NMA and his inability to be conciliatory strained their relations on a number of occasions.[2] The Association continued to nurse an animosity towards him even in his retirement. He was the only Past President of the Association never to be accorded a Past President's Pin when this honour was extended only from the immediate past incumbent, to all the living past presidents. McGrath never could accept, as Miller did, that the NMA had to act as the trade union for doctors, and government had to adapt to this fact.

It is not clear what particular measures McGrath and Miller hoped to push through with McGrath as Minister of Health. His eleven years in office was a period of extensive renovations to the General Hospital and an increase in the number of hospital beds in the province. It was also the period of mass immunization against poliomyelitis and measles, and from 1963 onwards of bursaries for premedical and predental students. It also saw the mandatory addition of Vitamin C to evaporated milk. All in all, it appears to have been a period of solid if unsensational achievements. But the public did not see it this way, neither did Miller. There was widespread dissatisfaction with the Department of Health which was perceived as doing nothing. As mentioned previously Miller was also concerned that services were deteriorating.[3]

In September 1967 McGrath, who had been in failing health for some years, was transferred from Health to Finance (Finance was considered the easiest Cabinet post, because Smallwood was the de facto Minister). The new Minister was John C. Crosbie. Relations between Miller and Crosbie were never warm and there was always a certain distance between the two . "We never did have the type of relationship that I had with other Ministers before him or after."[1] Miller ascribes this to the inability of Crosbie "to develop confidence in the people with whom he worked."[1] In other words Crosbie did not trust the officials of his own department for unbiased comprehensive briefing. It would follow that he would be tempted to seek elsewhere the enlightenment he was not able to find in his own department. This is what he was rumored to be doing. At least one of his confidants was said to be critical of Miller and this could only have added to his doubts about the reliability of his official advisors to provide impartial information.

Crosbie also feared that because Miller had been around so long he might have become out of date, and because of his age and health he was finding it difficult to measure up to the demands of the job. In spite of these misgivings Crosbie was fully aware of Miller's many estimable qualities and experience, he was "an invaluable resource knowing every physician in the province."

There was another trait of Crosbie's which must have been an irritation to Miller. To Miller, the Minister was responsible for the formulation and initiation of policy and should not concern himself with administrative details unless the Deputy Minister bought them to his attention. Crosbie seems to have interpreted his ministerial responsibilities as spilling into areas which Miller thought were his own domain. In a memo addressed to Miller and several other officials in the Department of Health[4] the Minister stated he wished 1) to be kept informed whenever a salaried physician resigned and the reasons and 2) disputes about salary or working conditions were to be discussed with the Minister before final decision by the department. Then the memo went on to say: "I wish to be kept informed in all cases where there is a possibility of friction between any member of the medical profession and the department." There is no record of Miller's response to this unfortunate memorandum which shows the Minister's lack of trust in his Deputy to bring to his attention all issues which might have repercussions. Miller may well have resented the memo addressed to him going to three other junior members of his department at the same time. If the Minister had thought such a memo necessary, it should have gone to Miller only, with instructions to notify his subordinates of the Minister's wishes. Still, Miller is generous in his praise of Crosbie and gives him full credit for drafting the complicated and time consuming legislation for medicare and seeing it through the legislature .

When Crosbie took over the Department of Health, there were two pressing issues on the agenda. The first was medicare. Originally it was slated to come in on 1 July 1968, but because of economic constraints it was postponed to 1 April 1969. It has been said that one of the reasons for replacing the Minister of Health was that the Department of Health had been dilatory in preparing for medicare. As we have seen (Chap. 10), Miller's many memoranda of this time, do not support the charge. The other pressing issue was the Medical School of which, as we have seen, the government was having second thoughts but of which Miller thought it was too late to backtrack.

Fortunately for both men, Crosbie was Minister for only seven months and was replaced by T.A. Hickman in May 1968 who also continued to hold the portfolio of Justice. Relations were warmer than with his predecessor . "He was a good Minister, easy to get along with, we didn't always agree – and we had an opportunity to discuss the things over which we did disagree." [1] Hickman describes Miller as " the perfect Deputy Minister". On Hickman's first day as Minister, Miller came into his office and in words which the Minister still remembers said, "I ought to outline to you my concept of my role. My role is to bring policies to your attention which you can reject, but I must continue to bring them to you. It is also my responsibility to advise against a course of action which in my view is not in the best interest of the department or government. If you reject my advice and embark on a policy with which I disagree I have an obligation without question to defend and implement that policy with enthusiasm." Miller was true to his word.

One of Hickman's tasks was the implementation of medicare. Of major concern was what the Cottage Hospital physicians would elect to do. The firm of consultants KPM proposed that every effort be made to keep the Cottage Hospitals' doctors on salary, by providing generous increases and other perks, but should a Cottage

Hospital physician choose to go fee for service, he would lose hospital privileges. Miller supported this proposal, except for the loss of hospital privileges. As he very sensibly pointed out to the minister, if all the salaried doctors in a locality opted to go for "fee for service", how could the Cottage Hospital be kept open? The Minister chose to follow the suggestion of KPM and began negotiations along these lines with the NMA which was acting as negotiator on behalf of the Cottage Hospital doctors. At a meeting between the NMA executive and the department, Miller, to Hickman's surprise, vigorously and cogently defended the Minister's position on loss of hospital privileges for Cottage Hospital physicians opting for fee for service. As he was leaving the room the Minister was accosted by the President of the NMA . "I know you're not enthusiastic about this proposal; [loss of Cottage Hospital privilege] it is Miller's idea." "No," said the Minister, "It was my idea."

Miller showed his wisdom in another incident relating to the implementation of medicare. To persuade people to register, the government proposed a massive advertising campaign and if that failed, a door to door campaign. Miller, practical and conscious of costs, proposed scrapping the former because if it did fail, a large sum of money would have been wasted.

The other business demanding the Minister's attention concerned the appointment of a Board for the General Hospital. Miller pointed out that Smallwood's expansion grants to the Grace and St. Clare's hospitals had left the General feeling bypassed. An Act had been passed to set up a corporation to run the hospital as demanded by the Canadian Hospital Association, but the Act had not been proclaimed. Miller pointed out that morale was bad in the hospital and would remain so until the Corporation was appointed. Hickman proposed getting Cabinet consent to the proclamation of the Act. Miller smiled. "Mr. Minister, I will give you the Victoria Cross if you can do that. Let me remind you, the General Hospital is the biggest source of political patronage in Newfoundland. I can tell you that Smallwood and his friends are not going to give that up." It soon became obvious to Hickman that Miller was right. Hickman repeatedly brought the matter up before the Cabinet, but Smallwood kept stalling. At this point an article appeared in a St. John's newspaper denouncing conditions at the General and warning that it was in danger of losing accreditation. The Cabinet was aghast. Hickman explained the crucial importance of accreditation. The Cabinet had no choice but to proclaim the Act.

The last Minister under whom Miller served, was Edward Roberts. Miller was a contemporary of his father but in spite of their age gap "after a few weeks we got along extremely well."[1] Roberts in turn had the highest confidence in Miller. "As a young Minister, I could not have had a better mentor. He had a wonderful sense of humor and could laugh at himself. He did not spend a lot of time on writing pieces of paper. He had been around so long – a walking legend. He had designed and built the system." Miller was pragmatic. Patients must be and would be taken care of, no matter what harebrained scheme the government might take up. When he heard of some impractical Cabinet plan for saving money, he would say to the Minister, "I don't care what the Cabinet does, the patients at the General must and are going to get three meals a day." While Miller was never tired of reminding the Minister that the running of the department was, by law, the Deputy Minister's responsibility,* he was careful to alert the Minister to incidents that could blow up into public scandals. Did Miller have any faults? According to Roberts, apart from his handwriting scrawl what faults he had stemmed from having been around so long. He did not tolerate fools gladly, or senseless comments. His views had become settled and his mind perhaps less open to new ideas. Certainly Roberts noticed no decline in physical or mental powers. "He worked long hours and effectively. I hear no complaints about people not being able to see him or getting the brush-off."

Miller and Smallwood

Smallwood had a high opinion of Miller describing him with his usual love of the superlative as "the incomparable Dr. Miller."[5] He paid a glowing tribute to him in the Legislature upon his retirement; a most unusual honour for a Deputy Minister.

Smallwood was Miller's senior by six years. Their acquaintance went back to the days when both men attended the sessions at the Methodist College Literary Institute. During the days of Commission of Government, they must have run into each other frequently

*"The Department of Health shall be administered by the Deputy Minister, assisted by one or more registered medical practitioners".

because Miller's Radio Health broadcasts and Smallwood's 'The Barrelman' followed each other. But they were never intimate, and treated each other formally and were never on first-name terms. In his memoir Miller perhaps understates the case when he said he "did not find [Smallwood] a difficult person to work with"[1] and adds, "The only serious disagreement I had with the Premier was over the proposed Children's Hospital." Still, when Miller was asked during his retirement if he still kept in touch with "Joey" he answered, "No, I saw too much of him in days gone by." The reason is not hard to guess. Smallwood's impulsive actions and antics were in stark contrast to Miller's carefully thought out practices and were a cause of frequent frustration to Miller. They sometimes made him cringe. In Smallwood's day, his office was linked to those of all his Ministers and Deputy Ministers through an intercom system. By pressing a button the Premier could bellow forth to anyone unfortunate enough to be at the other end of the line. Usually the occasions for such communications were precipitated by a visitor or delegation to the Premier's office with a request. Smallwood would rapidly decide which department should deal with the request, press the appropriate button and issue orders from the speaker on the wall (known as 'Joey's Squawk Boxes') to the official he had decided must to attend to the matter. A visitor to Miller's office remembers being startled to hear the well-known voice booming from the sqawk box, preposterous orders to Miller and Miller patiently trying to explain to the Premier why he could not dictate to a private hospital what it should do.

Smallwood's vision of himself as the defender of the little man and the champion of the poor, the one who saw that they got justice, added to his officials' workload. Everyone was encouraged to bring their complaints to the Premier's notice. Smallwood received a steady stream of letters and visitors asking for his help and in each case he would dictate a letter to the official whom he had chosen to attend to the petition; woe betide him if he passed the letter on to a more junior official, for Smallwood had issued strict orders through the clerk of the Executive Council, J. Channing, that the person designated in his letter was the one who must attend to the request. Miller had his share of petty complaints to attend to, passed his way by the Premier.

Like so many of his other activities, Smallwood's forays into the health field were for the showy and the spectacular, above all for votes. He loved nothing more than to be invited to lay the foundation stone of a new hospital or to preside at its opening. These occasions were opportunities for winning votes. It would be politically inept to pass them up. On one occasion he omitted the elementary precaution of finding out what it was he was supposed to be opening. It was enough that it had to do with health. He could depend on a timely briefing on arrival at the ceremony. On being enlightened, he said in disgust, "Why am I wasting my time here? There are no votes in a morgue".

It was over hospital construction that Smallwood caused most annoyance to the Department of Health. Public Works was responsible for these activities, but Health was expected to find the staff and operating funds for new or expanded hospitals that Smallwood had announced without any consultation with the Department of Health. Smallwood's disregard of the most elementary of financial considerations was amazing.

Smallwood had given a promise to enlarge the Springdale Hospital. The years passed and nothing happened. Finally, in 1968 the Springdale Chamber of Commerce reminded Smallwood of his promise.[6] Miller believed a promise must be kept and set in motion its execution. On another occasion, Smallwood was to lay the cornerstone of a new hospital. During lunch before the ceremony with guests, architect and contractors, Smallwood was carried away by his own exuberance and without any thought, announced that he was adding 30 beds to the number originally planned and grandiloquently confirmed the increase to the acclaiming crowd at the cornerstone laying ceremony. Smallwood could be intoxicated by an enthusiastic audience and make all sorts of rash promises. Two mining companies in Labrador City offered to build a new hospital. Smallwood, with his eye on the popular vote, had it built instead by the government with the help of donations from the companies. In the end he, for some unexplained reason, turned it over to the Salvation Army to run, a much more costly venture.

Towards the end of the Smallwood era Miller seems to have become uneasy about the haphazarded approach to hospital construction and renovations which he summed up in a long memorandum as follows:

> Practically all of the items [construction programs] deal with curative facilities and when completed would involve large increases in current expenditure. In recent years cost of construction and operating new facilities . . . has diminished emphasis on Public Health and Preventive Medicine to provide a well balanced health service.[7]

He then listed the construction programs under way or to which the government had made commitments, and warned, "Looking [at this list], it appears to me to be somewhat futile to continue [with this haphazard construction program] for another two years."[7] What Miller alluded to was that the Smallwood government was in dire financial straits and was looking for excuses to get out of rash, ill-considered commitments. He stressed the need "to establish some priorities and degrees of urgency" for the projects and the estimated cost of each. He was careful not to say which ones should be proceeded with and which ones dropped. That was a Ministerial or Cabinet decision, to be arrived at hopefully by "tailoring the suit to meet the cloth."

Political Pressure, Patronage and Payoffs

Political pressure is something all civil servants experience at one time or another. As related earlier, Miller first encountered it as a young doctor on the Labrador boat in 1930. But if Miller stuck to his guns on a matter of principal he also knew when to be pliable when no moral principal was at stake. An employee of the Department of Health with political influence had been caught stealing government supplies.[1] The department confronted him with his misdemeanor and initiated proceedings to get rid of him. Just then Miller had a call from Smallwood saying that while he didn't want to suggest sparing the employee, but would the department stay the proceedings until after the upcoming election? Miller agreed, but was intrigued by Smallwood's request. "'I'm sure that you don't need the few votes dependent on this man's job.' I shall never forget his answer. 'Doctor, a politician never has too many votes.'" Apart from these two somewhat innocuous examples, Miller related no other instances that could be construed as improper pressure. It is to

Smallwood's credit that he took over an excellent civil service and saw that its high standards were maintained.

One aspect of the Department of Health which Miller must have found unpleasant was patronage. During Commission of Government opportunities for patronage, if not vanished, were certainly limited. In his memoir, Miller mentions that Sir John Puddester was convinced that "it was better for him to look after his political friends," and then goes on to say that "at times it was difficult for those working there." [1] What these enigmatic phrases mean is not obvious, but the fairest construction to put on them is that under the Commission of Government, Puddester's ability to reward friends was still present, if curtailed. Patronage returned with a vengeance when Smallwood assumed office. It was particularly rampant in appointments to the support staff of the government-owned hospitals. Indeed, in the days of James McGrath it was said that any young person from his district of St. Mary's, was assured of a job at the General Hospital or at the Hospital for Mental and Nervous Diseases. But even he felt he must exercise a degree of restraint. On one occasion a physician at the Hospital for Mental and Nervous Diseases advertised for a technician. By far the best qualified applicant happened to come from St. Mary's Bay. The physician was told his choice was vetoed because the Minister said he had already appointed enough people from St. Mary's for the time being and if he were seen to favour any more it might have political repercussions. The physician passed the word on to Miller that the applicant from St. Mary's was by far the best qualified and the Minister would have to swallow his squeamishness and confirm the appointment, which McGrath did, but with reluctance.

Miller believed it was the prerogative of government to appoint whom it wished as long as it was made clear to those who got jobs through political influence that thenceforth they were on their own and should they be dismissed because of incompetence, dishonesty or some other valid reason, their benefactors would not lift a finger on their behalf. Miller was able to live with this type of patronage because generally the government abided by the rules of the game and did not intervene if the department dismissed an employee on good grounds. The lines were clearly drawn and each stayed onside.

Opportunities for patronage became more limited when the procedure for processing applications to the support staff of government-owned hospitals were promulgated. Politicians could submit names, but the final choice rested with a committee.[8] In spite of this safeguard, political appointments were still made. Doctor X who had served on a selection board had been outraged to find that an applicant other than the one recommended by the board had been appointed to a position through political influence. What chiefly annoyed Dr. X was not the appointment, but the farce of going through the motions of impartial selection then having it upset by a blatantly political choice. Dr. X felt his time was too valuable to be wasted on such charades. Miller's somewhat lame comment on the incident was "Dr. X is realistic in his outlook and is well aware that there are complicating factors in some appointments."[9]

If Miller had learned to accept patronage as a fact of life he must have found pay-offs and kick-backs extremely distasteful. Under the Smallwood regime, a deplorably corrupt system grew up in the purchase of supplies for the Department of Health.* Contracts for supplies were awarded without tender or on the understanding that the price would "be adjusted later," that is, go up in a few weeks. Miller accepted the right of the Government to buy where it wished, but that was all. Miller was scrupulously honest and never enriched himself from the public till. Once he was negotiating with the representative of a pharmaceutical firm for the bulk purchase of a drug. The arrangements concluded, the representative asked, "What percent shall I add on top, Dr. Miller?" Miller was astounded and said, "Nothing." Commenting on the incident later to his son he said, "I don't know what goes on in ____ but obviously they take a slice off the top for themselves."

He strove to stop kick-backs, but could only succeed by indirect methods. Once when Dr. Ian Rusted, Consultant Internist to the Government, was visiting a Cottage Hospital, he observed an expensive brand of a medication on a shelf in the dispensary. On his return he told Miller, who recommended that he tour the Division of Central Supplies, and make recommendations. He found many unnecessarily expensive brands of medications. Rusted recommended to Miller that in future all medications be bought on tender. Miller

* Supplies were purchased by the Government Purchasing Agency upon request from the Department of Health and stocked in the latter's Division of Central Supplies.

passed on this recommendation with his own endorsement and it was adopted, but not without protest.

Kick-backs were impossible in federal-funded programs. By the end of Miller's career when tenders had become the practice for provincial contracts, kick-backs, at least in their most blatant forms, had been eliminated.

Miller, as the chief civil servant in his department for so many years, was called upon to serve under eight Commissioners or Ministers, each with a different personality and conception of his role as head of the department. Naturally Miller preferred some to others and as was bound to happen, disagreements arose from time to time, but these were never permitted to disrupt the smooth functioning of the department. Much of the credit for this happy state of affairs must go to Miller but also to the good sense of the Ministers themselves. Still, their relations with Miller must have been constrained by the realization that this was no ordinary civil servant, but one who had attained an extraordinary prestige early in his career and who also enjoyed the confidence of Smallwood.

Chapter 22 – Notes

1. NRC Miller, L.A. Memoir, Unpublished.

2. McGrath, J. "*Casual Memories From Half a Century of Medical Practice in Newfoundland.*" Newfoundland Medical Association Newsletter. 16:9-11-1974.

3. IRC LAM to JMcG 1959-10-5.

4. CNS JCCC JCC to LAM, TAK, WPC, and TS, 1968-01-18.

5. Smallwood, JR ibid p. 378.

6. CNS JCCC JDW to JCC 1968-01-20.

7. CNS JCCC LAM to JCC 1967-11-07.

8. CNS Memorandum Department of Health 1967-11-17.

9. CNS EMRC LAM Comments on Memorandum of CJG to Cottage Hospital Secretaries and Nurses, 1970-09-14.

CHAPTER 23

Epilogue

In 1958, at the height of his career, in a speech to the St. John's Rotary Club, Miller took time to take stock of the strides in health care that had occurred in his lifetime.[1] Always modest, he said nothing about his role in bringing them about. The spectacular drop in mortality and infectious disease rates, the cottage hospital scheme, the only government-sponsored health care plan of its kind in Canada, were all sources of gratification. He put in his usual plea for more hospital beds for the acutely and mentally ill. Then Miller posed the question "whither are we tending?" He proceeded to give a series of predictions. It is a revealing list showing the things he wanted to happen or to correct, the wrong prognostications and failure to foresee what did occur. To single out the more important: dental caries would disappear; all babies would be born in hospitals*; rehabilitation and vocational guidance services would be available. He would have been wiser not to have predicted that the cause of cancer would be found in the next quarter century or that the population of the province would plateau off at seven hundred and fifty thousand. Like many others Miller appears to have failed to foresee two significant developments in the near future and their consequences – the drop in the birth rate and the end of the post war boom. But he can be forgiven for being no more perspicacious than the rest of his contemporaries.

* The practice of midwifery had been regulated by an act of the Commission of Government.[2] After 1959 no new midwife licences were issued except to the nurse-midwives of the IGA. [3]

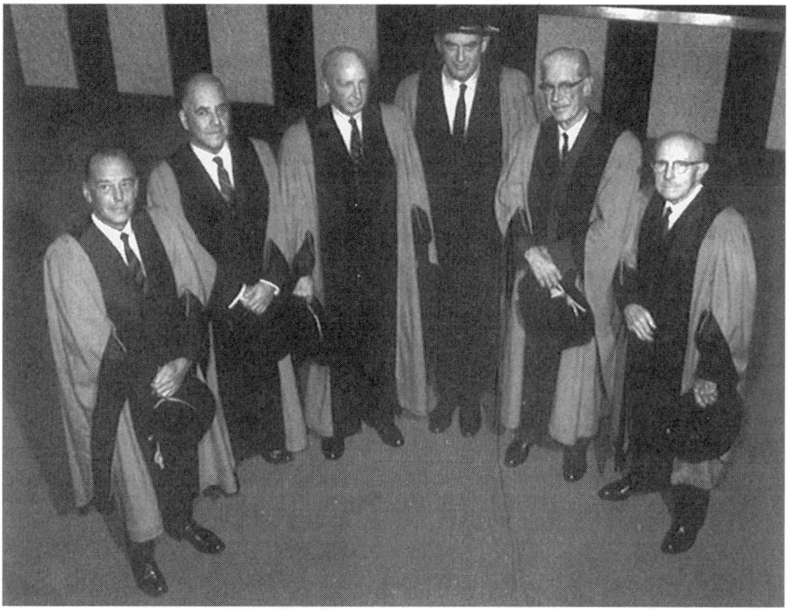

Leonard in Good Company

Doctor of Laws (Honoris Causa) Dalhousie University 1968 on the occasion of the centennial of the first faculty of medicine at the university. (left to right.) Dr. Harold Ernest Taylor, professor of pathology at the University of British Columbia; Dr Leonard Miller; Dr. Ronald Ian Macdonald, associate dean and professor of medicine, University of Toronto; Sir Peter Medawar, eminent British researcher, Dr. C.J. Beckwith, executive secretary of the Nova Scotia Medical Society; Dr. Clyde Wallace Holland, Halifax.

Courtesy Dalhousie Medical School

In June 1971 having reached the statutory retirement age of sixty-five, he retired. In spite of his gloomy forebodings, uttered on a number of occasions, the health services of the province had not deteriorated and perhaps were in as healthy a state as they were ever to be.

The occasion of his retirement was marked by tributes on the floor of the Legislature, an unheard of compliment for a retiring Deputy Minister. Premier Smallwood's words sum up the feelings of the province which he had served so faithfully and competently for so long. "It is with a sense of deep gratitude that I inform the House of the impending retirement of a devoted and faithful public servant."[4] Public recognition of Miller's achievements had begun to appear in the years just before his retirement. Two deserve particular notice. In October 1971 he was granted the Degree of Doctor of

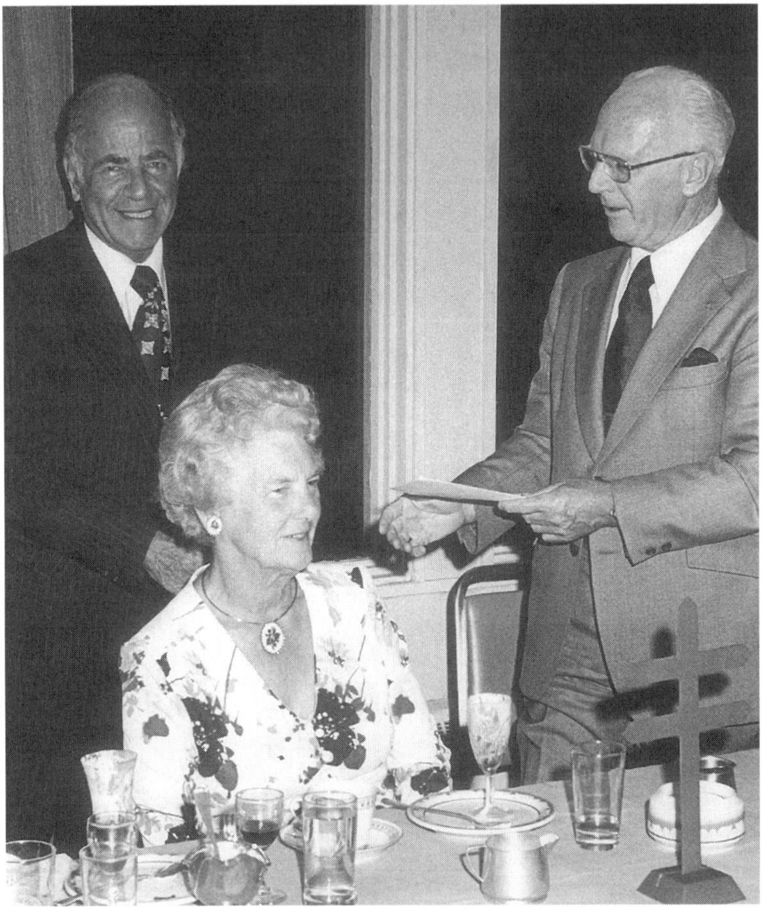

Recognition 1971, Honorary President Newfoundland Tuberculosis Association. Leonard, Myra and Edgar House. (Courtesy Mrs Lorraine Balderson.)

Science (Honoris Causa) by Memorial University. In presenting him for the degree, the Public Orator, Dr. George Story, used these words: "He has served and directed the largest of all Government Departments and played a signal role in one of the most critical of all the revolutions in Newfoundland's history . . . at the University we have known him as the warm friend of our Medical School, but all Newfoundlanders know him as the modest, selfless administrator of the Health Services who may say as he retires in Othello's plain words, 'I have done the state some service.'" No better words could have been chosen to characterize Miller's career.

In December 1979, the old General Hospital, now a chronic care institution, was renamed The Leonard Miller Centre. Never before or since has a health care facility been named after a civil servant.

During the years left to him, Miller sat on the boards of a number of voluntary organizations where his presence was invaluable because of his detailed knowledge of the workings of government. He had developed ischemic heart disease about the time of his retirement and spent the winters in Florida. He died on 5 December 1981 aged seventy-five.

Looking back at a career which to others appears so successful, Miller did not think he could afford to be quite so self-congratulatory. He lamented that he had not been more successful in persuading the public and the government that prevention was better than cure; to direct more resources into public health and less into "curative medicine". The other failure of his professional career, he thought, was the lack of long-term planning.[5] But Miller need not shoulder responsibility for these two "failures". In his day the clamour was for more and bigger hospitals and the expensive equipment and technology that went with them. These were the pressures to which governments had to bow . From his very earliest days Miller had been an advocate of public health. This was where his interest lay. He repeatedly warned governments and the public of the error of too much emphasis on treatment rather than preventing illness and the folly of neglecting long-term planning. But long-term planning was unattainable while Smallwood was at the helm and perhaps is too subject to unforeseen circumstances ever to be more than an aspiration. Whether Miller could have done more to remedy the unbalanced policies of his era can only be a subject of speculation. He did all he could and in his old age he shouldered the blame for the consequences of his warnings falling on deaf ears.

Some years after his retirement he was visiting the Centre which bears his name. On the elevator he told the operator at which floor he wished to get off . The operator shot past his floor to let the other passengers off first. As the elevator descended to Miller's floor, the operator apologized to Miller saying, "We must take care of our doctor's first."

Chapter 23 – Notes

1. The St. John's Evening Telegram 1958 -02-12.

2. PANL GN 38 S1-1-2 An Act To Govern the Practice of Midwifery 1936.

3. Lewis J. Personal Communication.

4. The St. John's Evening Telegram 1971-04-14.

5. IRC Miller, L.A *The Need for Planning*, (Speech to the Newfoundland Hospital Association). 1972-10- 16 . Unpublished.

Bibliography

Adams, Ian, *The Poverty War*. McClelland & Stewart Ltd. Toronto.

Brown, Cassie, *A Winter's Tale, The Wreck of the Florizel.* Doubleday Canada Ltd. Toronto Ontario, 1976.

Bassler, Gerhard P, *Sanctuary Denied.* Published by the Institute of Social and Economic Research Memorial University of Newfoundland, 1992.

Encyclopedia of Newfoundland and Labrador. Vol. 7. 1991 Harry Cuff Publicating Ltd. St. John's, Newfoundland.

Gwyn, R.G. *Smallwood the Unlikely Revolutionary.* McCelland and Stewart Ltd., Toronto Canada, 1968.

Hiller, James and Neary, Peter (Editors) *Twentieth Century Newfoundland Explorations*: Breakwater, St. John's, NF AlC 6E6, 1994.

Kahn, Alison. *Listen While I Tell You.* Institute of Social and Economic Research, Memorial University of Newfoundland, 1987.

Lewis, J. Shrimpton M. *Notes Towards an Assessment of Health Policy under Commission of Government* (unpublished).

Leyton, Elliott *Dying Hard. The Ravages of Industrial Carnage* McCelland and Stewart Ltd., Toronto.

McCorquodale S. *Public Administration in Newfoundland During the Period of Commission of Government: A question of Political Development* (Ph.D. Thesis Queen's University 1973) (unpublished) CNS.

Medjuck, S. *Jews of Atlantic Canada.* Breakwater Books, St. John's, NF, 1986.

Miller, L.A., Unpublished Memoir, 39 pages, Undated 1978?, courtesy of Dr. Nigel Rusted

Newfoundland Royal Commission HM Stationery Office Kingsway London, 1933.

Noel, S.J.R. *Politics in Newfoundland.* University of Toronto Press. Toronto and Buffalo, 1971.

O'Brien, Patricia. *Out of Sight. A History of the Waterford Hospital.* Breakwater Books, 277 Duckworth St., St. John's, NF AlC 6E6, 1989.

Roberts, C.A. *From Fishing Cove to Faculty Council.* Pondhead Publishers. Calgary, Alberta Canada, 1995.

Rompkey, Ronald *Grenfell of Labrador. A Biography.* University of Toronto Press, Toronto, Buffalo, London, 1991.

Rusted, Nigel. *The Devil Deep Down There.* Faculty of Medicine, Memorial University of Newfoundland, 1981.

Saunders, Gary L. *Doctor Olds of Twillingate.* Portrait of an American Surgeon in Newfoundland. Breakwater Books, St. John's, NF, 1994.

Smallwood, Joseph, R. *I Chose Canada.* MacMillan and Company of Canada, 1977.

Thomas, Gordon W. *From Sled to Satellite – My Years in the Grenfell Mission.* Irwin Publishing Inc. Printed in Canada by John Deyell Co, 1987.

Appendix

Appendix I

Chronology

1906	– Born in St. John's, NF
1912	– Death of mother
1918	– Father drowned on *The Florizel*
1926	– B.A. Dalhousie University, NS. Internship: Victoria General Hospital, Halifax, NS
1930	– M.D. C.M. - Dalhousie University
1930	– 1934 - General practice St. John's, NF
1933	– Part-time MHO
1933	– Marries Myra Chafe of Brigus, NF
1933-34	– Postgraduate studies in pediatrics in Vienna
1934	– Full-time MHO
1934	– Birth of daughter Lorraine (Balderson)
1935-36	– Rockefeller Fellowship, Harvard School of Public Health, Certificate in Public Health
1937	– Birth of son Keith
1939	– MPH Harvard
1942-45	– Civil Defence Volunteer
1944	– Director of Medical Services
1949	– Deputy Minister of Health ,Newfoundland

1950 & 1964 – Member of Canadian Delegation to World Health Organization

1967 – President Canadian Public Health Association

1967 – Centennial Medal

1968 – Doctor of Laws (Honoris Causa) Dalhousie University

1971 – Retires

1971 – Doctor of Science (Honoris Causa) Memorial University of Newfoundland

1972-74 – Royal Commission on Nursing Education, Newfoundland

1978 – 25th. Anniversary Elizabeth II Medal

1978 – Companion, Order of Canada

1979 – Former General Hospital renamed the Leonard Miller Centre

1981 – Death

Associations, Club Memberships and Awards

Past President St. John's Clinical Society of Newfoundland

Past President Newfoundland Medical Association

Past President Canadian Public Health Association

Past President St. John's Kinsmen Club

Past Master Masonic Lodge Tasker

Honorary Member Canadian Lung Association

Director International Grenfell Association

1936 Member Beta Chapter Delta Omega Society

1939 Honorary Life Member St. John Ambulance Association

1951 Royal College of Physicians and Surgeons of Canada. Certificate in Public Health (Honorary)

1965 Honorary Member Canadian Red Cross Newfoundland Division

1968 Golden Anniversary Award Canadian National Institute for the Blind

1970 Honorary Membership Association of Registered Nurses of Newfoundland

1971 Citizen of The Year St. John's Junior Chamber of Commerce

1971 Citation of Merit Canadian Cancer Society, Newfoundland Division

1971 Life Member Newfoundland Medical Association

1971 Honorary President Newfoundland Tuberculosis Association

1972 Honorary Life Membership Newfoundland Hospital Association

1972 Honorary Life Member Newfoundland Dental Society

1973 Senior Member Canadian Medical Association.

1973-1975 Honorary Chairman - Christmas Seal Campaign

Appendix II

People Interviewed

Ayre, Olga	Child Welfare Association
Balderson, Jeffrey	Grandson
Balderson, Kenneth	Grandson
Balderson, Lorraine	Daughter
Blanchard, T.A.	Secretary, Royal Commission on Health
Brooks, Yvette	First Cousin
Burnell, Robin	Department of Health
Chalker, The Hon. J.R.	Minister of Health
Clift, Shannon	Contemporary
Clouston, A.	Kinsmen's Club
Coates, R.	Secretary 1948 - 1955
Crosbie, The Hon. J.C.	Minister of Health
Eaton, Douglas	Medical School
Feder, H.	Jewish Community
Galway, Cyril	Department of Health
Godden, Phyllis, RN	Child Welfare Association
Hennebury, Sister Fabian	St. Clare's Hospital
Hickman, Mr. Justice T.A.	Minister of Health
House, Daphne	Department of Health
House, Edgar	Newfoundland Tuberculosis Society
Kelland, D.	Department of Health
Kelly, Janet	Dr. J. McGrath (Father)
Lewis, Jean RN	Department of Health
McGrath, Elizabeth	Dr. J. McGrath (Father)
Miller, Edgar	Cousin
Miller, Keith	Son
Miller, Michael	Nephew
Morgan, M.	Medical School
Moores, Ralph	Department of Health

Munn, A.	Friend
Nevitt, Joyce, RN	Memorial University School of Nursing
Pearce, A.	Friend
Peters, Dr. D.	Dental Services
Roberts, E., QC	Minister of Health
Skirving, H.	Department of Health
Squires, Joan	Secretary, 1958 - 68 1970 - 71 1973 - 74
Story, J., RN	General Hospital
Thomas, Patricia	IGA
Wilansky, Maurice	Jewish Community

Physicians Interviewed or who communicated with the author.

Anderson, T
Collins, John
Coxon, M
Gray, Jean D.
Harley, Brian
Henderson, C.U.
Hollywood, Brian
House, Max
Josephson, J.
Knowling, A.
Knowling, Ethne
Lawton, L.
MacLaughlin, E.A.
Mercer, A.R.
Murphy, N.
Neville-Smith, C.
Parsons, W.D.
Roberts, Charles
Ross, John
Rowe, A.T.
Rusted, Ian
Rusted, Nigel
Severs, D.
Shapter, A.E.
Simms, Graham
Simms, R.
Simpson, Ian
Suttie, Boyd
Thomas, G.W.
Walsh, Cyril
Warrick, P.

Appendix III

Commission of Government
The Department of Public Health and Welfare 1934-1949

Commissioner	1934	John C. Puddester
Secretary		H.M. Mosdell
Director of Medical Services	1944	L.A. Miller
Commissioner	1947	H.W. Quinton

Province of Newfoundland
Department of Health 1949-1971

Minister of Health	1949	H.W. Quinton
	1949	J.R. Chalker
	1952	P.S. Forsey
	1954	S.J. Hefferton
	1956	J. McGrath
	1967	John C. Crosbie
	1968	T.A.J. Hickman
	1969	E. Roberts
Deputy Minister		L.A. Miller

Appendix IV

Articles by Leonard A. Miller*

Miller L. *A Plea for Public Health.* Nova Scotia Medical Bulledn 21:346-3501942.

Miller L.A. *The People, The Doctor and the State,* Presidential Address to NMA (Unpublished) 22 June 1943.

Miller L. *Public Health in Newfoundland.* Canadian Journal of Public Health 41 (1): 1-6 1950.

Miller L. *Public Health and Medical Care in Newfoundland.* Canadian Medical Association Journal 64 (1):52 -55 1951.

Miller L.A. *Spectacular Changes in Public Health Picture.* Newfoundland Journal of Commerce 25:49-51 1958.

Miller L. *The Newfoundland Department of Health* Canadian Journal of Public Health 50 (6): 228-39 1959.

Miller L. *The Children's Health Plan in Newfoundland.* Canadian Journal of Public Health 51 (10) :385-388 1960.

Miller L. *The Newfoundland Department of Health.* Federal and Provincial Health Services in Canada 1962.

Miller L. *History of Health Services.* Canadian Hospital 39 (2): 47 1962.

Miller L. *Cottage Hospital System.* Canadian Hospital 39 (2): 48-49 1962.

Miller L. *Medical Manpower in Newfoundland – A Preliminary Study.* Newfoundland Medical Association Newsletter 7 (4):8-10 1965.

Miller L.A. and Hatcher G.A. *Public Medical Care Programs in Newfoundland.* Canadian Journal Public Health 56: 69-73 1965.

Millcr L.A. *Medicare.* Newfoundland Journal Commerce 35 (2): 28-31, 38 1968.

Miller L.A. *The Need For Planning.* Address to the Newfoundland Hospital Association. Unpublished 16 October 1972.

Miller L. *The Cottage Hospital Plan in Newfoundland.* Newfoundland Medical Association Newsletter 16 (4): 23-27 1974.

* This is a minimum list. Miller left no list or copies of his articles.

Miller L. *British and Irish Contributions to Canadian Medicine.* Newfoundland Medical Association Newsletter 18 (6): 10-14 1976.

Miller Memoir 39 pages ?1978 (unpublished) Courtesy of Dr. Nigel Rusted.

Miller L.A. *History of Cottage Hospitals,* (address to Medical History Society 9 Oct. 1980) Unpublished.

Miller L. *Placement Incentives* (letter) Canadian Medical Association Journal 126 (2): 120 1982.

Abbreviations

ACMC	Association of Canadian Medical Colleges
AGM	Annual General Meeting of the Newfoundland Medical Association
ANLMA	Archives of Newfoundland and Labrador Medical Association
ARNN	Association of Registered Nurses of Newfoundland
BBC	British Broadcasting Company
BN	Bachelor of Nursing
CMA	Canadian Medical Association
CNS	Centre of Newfoundland Studies
DMS	Director of Medical Services
EMRC	Edward M. Roberts Collection
Ex Com	Executive Committee of the Newfoundland Medical Association
HSC	Health Sciences Centre
HRF	Health Resources Fund
IRC	Ian Rusted Collection
IGA	International Grenfell Association
JCCC	John C. Crosbie Collection
JRSC	Joseph R. Smallwood Collection
KPM	Kates Peat Marwick
MAC	Medical Advisory Council of the General Hospital
MAR	Newfoundland Department of Mines, Agriculture and Resources
MHO	Medical Health Officer
MPH	Master of Public Health
MUN	Memorial University of Newfoundland
NF	Newfoundland
NHGP	Federal National Health Grants Program

NH&W	Federal Department of National Health and Welfare
NMA	Newfoundland Medical Association (now Newfoundland & Labrador Medical Association)
NONIA	Newfoundland Outport Nursing and Industrial Association
NRC	Nigel Rusted Collection
NS	Nova Scotia
NTA	Newfoundland Tuberculosis Society
PANL	Provincial Archives of Newfoundland and Labrador
PH&W	Commission of Government Department of Public Health and Welfare
STD	Sexually Transmitted Diseases
RCMP	Royal Canadian Mounted Police
RN	Registered Nurse
RNMDSF	Royal National Mission to Deep Sea Fishermen
USP	U.S. Picture and Portrait Company
WDPC	W. David Parsons Collection

Names for Initials in References

ADM	Administrator
ARM	A.R. Mercer MD
BS	Boyd Suttie MD
CAS	C.A. Streets
CBS	C.B. Stewart MD
CHP	Charles H. Pottle MD
CJ	Charles Janeway MD
CJG	Cyril J. Galway
CKH	C.K. Howse
CSC	Charles S. Curtis MD
CUH	Charles U. Henderson MD
DB	D. Baird MD
DGB-W	D.G. Brett -Williams DDS

DP	D. Piper
DH	Douglas C. Hunt
EABW	E.A.B. Wilmer
EJP	E.J. Phelan
ESP	E.S. Peters MD
EP	Eric Pike MD
ER	E. Roberts QC
FWG	Frederick W. Jackson MD
GEC	George E. Cummings
GG	G. Gover
HJH	H.J. Hann DDS
HM	H. Mosdell MB
IR	Ian Rusted MD
JA Mac F	J.A. MacFarlane MD
JBR	James B. Roberts MD
JCC	John C. Crosbie QC
JCP	John Charles Puddester
JDW	J.D. Williamson
JEJ	J.E. Josephson MD
JMcG	James McGrath MB
JR	John Ross MB
JRC	J.R. Chalker
JRS	Joseph R.Smallwood
JWMcL	J. Wendell McLeod MD
LAM	Leonard Albert Miller MD
LED	L.E. Drake
LM	Leonard A. Martin
MOM	Moses Morgan
PJW	Pat J. Whelan MD
PSF	P.S. Forsey
PW	Philip Woods MB
RAD	R.A. Daniel
RG	Ray Gushue

RJB	R.J. Burnell
RQ	R. Quigley DDS
RSF	Robert S. Furlong
TAH	T. Alec Hickman
TAK	T. Arthur Knowling MB
TS	T. Sellars
WAP	W. Anthony Paddon MD
WDP	W. David Parsons MD
WLC	William L. Cochrane MD
WPC	William P. Collingwood MD
WRC	W.R. Callahan
WTG	Wilfred T. Grenfell MD (Hon.)

Index

Page references for photographs appear in bold.

I

J

K

L

M